Heidi Sze

Words and Recipes for the New Mother

Nurturing Your New Life

HarperCollins*Publishers*

IMPORTANT INFORMATION

While this book is intended as a general information resource and all care has been taken in compiling the contents, it does not take into account individual circumstances and individual needs and is not in any way rendering medical advice, nor should it be used as a substitute for medical, psychological or dietary advice. It is essential that you always seek advice as appropriate from a qualified health professional on all specific situations and conditions of concern. The author and publisher cannot be held responsible for any claim or action that may arise from reliance on the information contained in this book.

HarperCollins_Publishers_

First published in Australia in 2019
by HarperCollinsPublishers Australia Pty Limited
ABN 36 009 913 517
harpercollins.com.au

HarperCollins_Publishers_
Level 13, 201 Elizabeth Street, Sydney, NSW 2000, Australia
Unit D1, 63 Apollo Drive, Rosedale, Auckland 0632, New Zealand
A 53, Sector 57, Noida, UP, India
1 London Bridge Street, London, SE1 9GF, United Kingdom
Bay Adelaide Centre, East Tower, 22 Adelaide Street West, 41st Floor,
    Toronto, Ontario, M5H 4E3, Canada
195 Broadway, New York, NY 10007

A catalogue record for this book is available from the National Library of Australia

ISBN: 978 1 4607 5730 7 (paperback)
ISBN: 978 1 4607 1105 7 (ebook : epub)

Cover and internal design by Amy Daoud, HarperCollins Design Studio
Cover images courtesy of Heidi Sze
Layout and typesetting by Jane Waterhouse
All photographs are courtesy of Heidi Sze and her family, except as noted.
Photographs by Katherine Schultz Photography: pages iv, 3, 34–5, 58–9, 60, 67, 82, 96, 100, 116–17, 118, 154–5, 161, 192–3, 202, 206, 211, 224–5, 256–7, 263 and 265–305
Author photograph on page 258 by Tim Grey
Colour reproduction by Splitting Image Colour Studio, Clayton VIC
Printed and bound in China by RR Donnelley

For Joan, who made me a mother

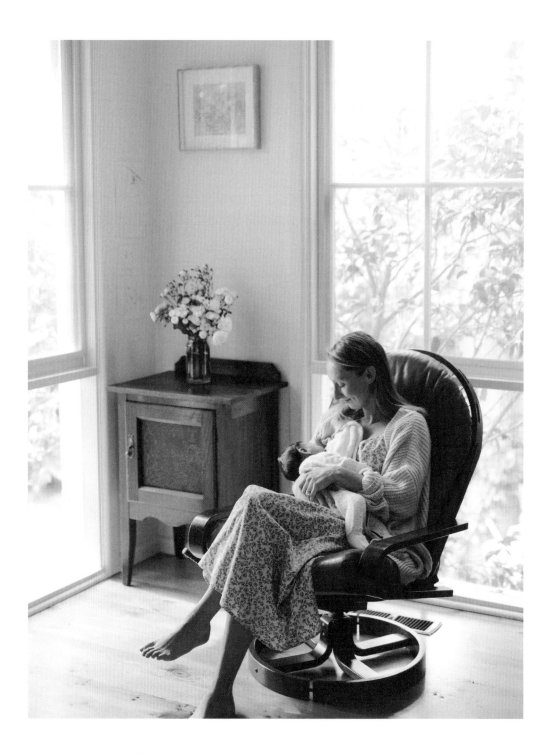

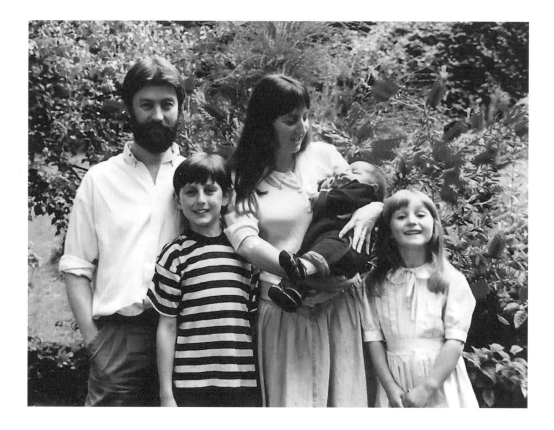

Introduction

When I was 5 years old, my mother gave birth to my younger brother. I remember the day well. We were at a birth centre in the city and my father, grandmother, older brother and I were in the room, along with a couple of midwives. People were moving swiftly, yet everything felt calm as our tiny new family member came into the world. Despite this clear snapshot of my brother's birth, I have few memories of his newborn days.

As I grew up, babies rarely crossed my path – at least not long enough to elaborate on my impression that they were cute, smelled curiously great and seemed to do very little besides feed and sleep.

When my husband, Ben, and I found out we were going to be parents, this was more or less what we were expecting. Beyond my insight as a dietitian that certain foods would be beneficial after birth, my knowledge about postnatal life was light and limited. And so we prepared in a way that many parents-to-be do in our present day and age – we bought stuff. By 15 weeks, I was deep in online pram reviews, and by 23 weeks the bassinet was delivered. Week by week, we ticked items off our list, so that by the time our baby was born we would have everything we needed, and we would be ready.

What I learned the night my daughter, Joan, galloped into the world was that the only thing she really needed was me. There are nifty creations that can make your life easier, but nothing can tame the primal need for contact and milk. Some infants require advanced medical care to thrive, and we are fortunate to live in a time when this is available. But generally speaking, the empowering and overwhelming truth is that babies only need you. They need you all day and sometimes all night, no matter how tired you are and with no regard for your modern-world obligations.

Matrescence, the process of becoming a mother, has always been a time of great change in a woman's life, but these days the transition feels even greater. Most of us aren't privy to the realities of motherhood, as we no longer live in close companionship with previous generations. While our species has evolved in many other ways, the needs of newborns and the mother–baby relationship remains intensely animalistic, a fact that isn't always acknowledged or supported – culturally or politically.

It's easy to see, then, why many of our expectations surrounding pregnancy and motherhood are unrealistic. Images of contented smiles, growing bellies and mothers seemingly carrying out the job with ease lead us to believe this is how our experience will and should be. Books on getting

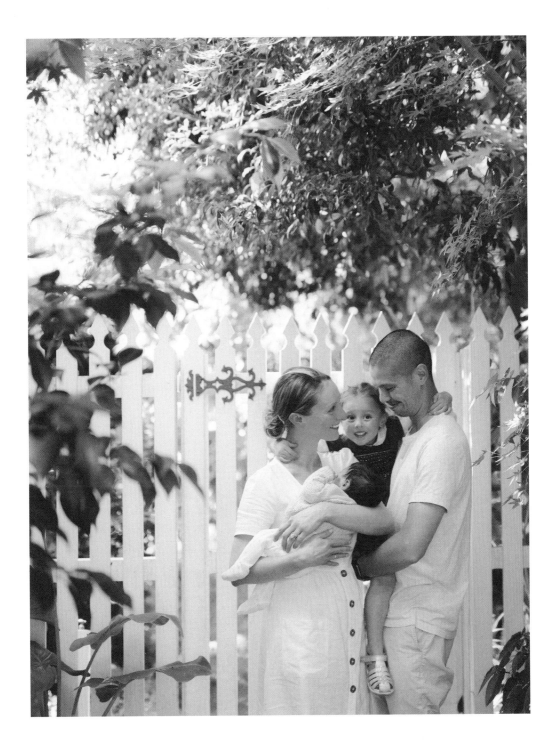

your baby to sleep through the night and fitting back into your pre-baby jeans lead vulnerable new mothers, and society at large, to believe this is what we should be aiming for, and that once these aims are achieved all will be well.

These unrealistic expectations are fuelled by a lack of transitional support for women who want to pause their careers to have a family, which feeds the assumption that we should be able to 'bounce back' after having a baby and 'do it all'. The reality is, no-one can do it all on their own; motherhood is a time of significant change and profound alteration to the way a woman thinks, feels and functions, and for most of us there will be no bouncing. Especially while we recover from pregnancy and childbirth, and settle in to our new lives.

No woman can prepare for motherhood completely, nor can we predict how our experience will unfold. Indeed, the entire process of conceiving, growing, birthing and caring for our children probably won't happen as we imagine. I, for one, never envisaged I would need to take medication to conceive my first child, nor that I would spend the first 18 weeks of that pregnancy gagging at the sight of vegetables. I also never imagined my baby would remain in a breech position until the end and that there would be talk of a c-section. It was when my waters broke at 38 weeks and I found myself, soon afterwards, breathing my breech baby down and out through my birth canal that I realised how wildly unpredictable my life had become, and how intense my emotions and experiences as a mother could be.

Once I began preparing for baby number two – a boy named Walt – I was able to appreciate that the best way to get ready for this impending life change is to accept the fact that it is going to be life changing, unpredictable and intense, and to make space for that. I could work on releasing my expectations and, instead, try to tune in to, and accept, my reality; I could put support systems in place that would allow me to focus on nurturing – because, for a while, that might be all I could manage; I could strive to offer myself compassion as I once again cared for a newborn baby, only now with a 3-year-old who also needed me; and I could surround myself with people who reminded me to do these things – who would ask me how I was feeling, tell me I was doing a wonderful job and offer me a sandwich.

To those of you entering into the season of new motherhood, my hope is that you will find recognition and reassurance here, in these pages. Bringing a baby into the world and guiding them through it requires you to give, surrender and grow in ways that may be inconceivable before becoming a mother.

It's hard work, glorious work. It's also hungry work. And though I may not be able to offer you a sandwich, I can give you a recipe and remind you to nourish and care for yourself, reverently and with abundance, as you set about nurturing your new life.

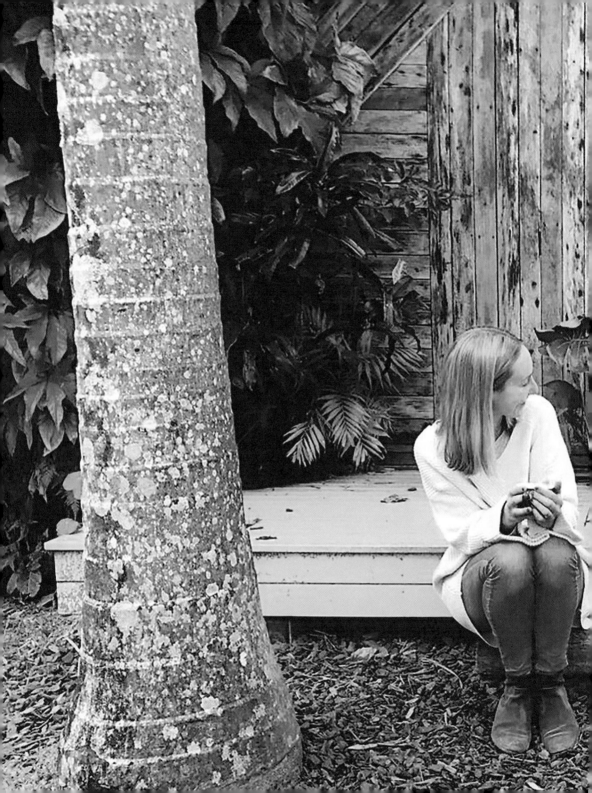

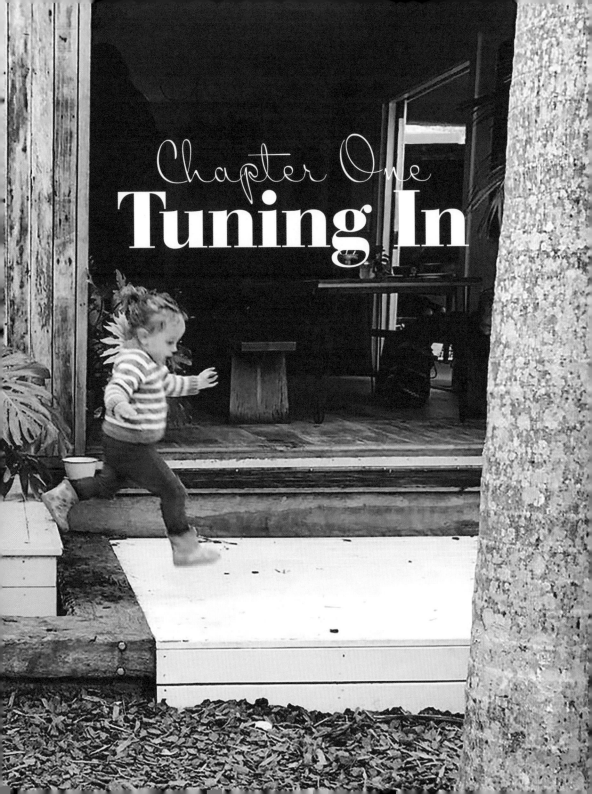

Chapter One

Tuning In

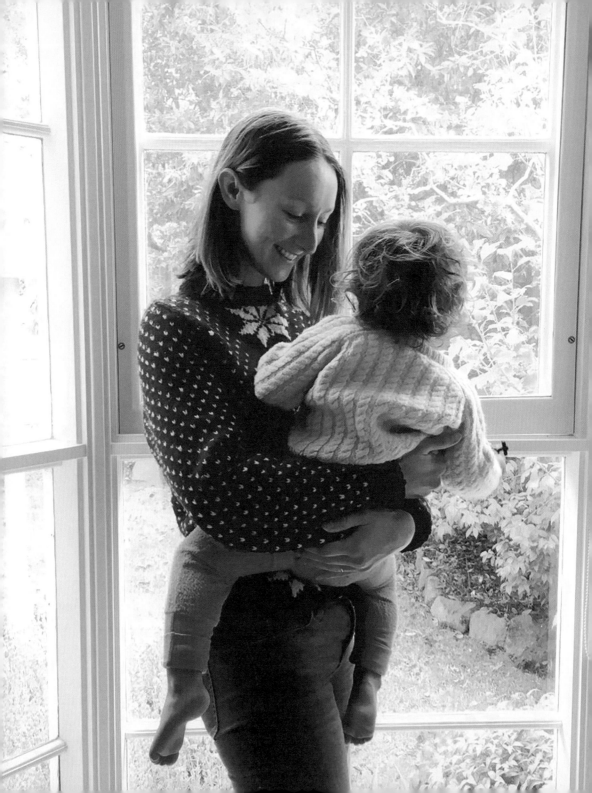

I knew my period wasn't going to come. It was due, and in the days leading up to its expected arrival I had experienced cramping on and off, which usually signals the beginning of my menstrual cycle. But something felt different from the previous two months Ben and I had spent trying to conceive our second child. Pregnancy and premenstrual symptoms are frustratingly similar, and so, as is often the case when making babies, I just had to wait and see.

In an attempt to cushion the blow were I not pregnant, I comforted myself with the fact that we hadn't been trying for long and most couples take many more months to conceive. Also, if this wasn't our month, it meant we'd likely be able to attend a family wedding in Hong Kong later that year. I repeated these things to myself, but with an underlying sense of certainty that I wouldn't be renewing my passport. And I was right, I was pregnant. But we did end up going on that trip. Because instead of leading to my second child, my second pregnancy led to my first miscarriage.

Miscarriage is a common and utterly devastating experience. Our loss, though heartbreaking, left me with a greater respect for my body's innate wisdom. Most early miscarriages are caused by chromosomal abnormalities and are a normal part of making healthy babies. I found comfort in surrendering to this fact and the sometimes wondrous, sometimes painful process of growing new life.

Nevertheless, it was unsettling to observe my intuition clash with my reality. You see, from the moment I suspected I was pregnant, I felt I was carrying a strong and healthy baby. It wasn't until my 8-week scan, as my obstetrician spent far too long searching for a heartbeat, that I felt differently. I wondered, had I not attended that appointment and carried on assuming I was pregnant for a few more weeks, would my initial feeling have changed? Would I have noticed something was off, as my body prepared to release and reset? After resting on the couch while crying for my lost baby with a hot water bottle down my pants (miscarriage really is a shitty, shitty thing), I came to understand that it didn't matter either way.

So often in life, when we open ourselves up to receive good and valuable experiences, we must make ourselves vulnerable to heartache. Tuning in doesn't alter this fact; it can't help us to foresee outcomes and protect ourselves from pain. Rather, being in tune with who we are and how we are feeling helps us to know what we need in order to continue allowing ourselves to be open and vulnerable. To keep going through it all. If 'tuning in' sounds vague to you, don't worry, I get it. This kind of language can seem a bit hippy-dippy, so let's make things clear. Tuning in simply means knowing who you are and paying attention to how you are feeling. While that may sound simple enough, in our present culture, many of us are unfamiliar with the practice.

From a young age, we are flooded with external influences that inform our beliefs on who we should be, what we should want, how we should spend our money, what we should weigh, what we should eat, when we should be working, when we should be making babies and how we should raise them. It can, therefore, feel foreign to look within, and yet it serves us greatly to do so.

Tuning in connects us to our inner self – that is, who we are at our core, what our values are and how we tick. These are essential things to know if we wish to live a fulfilling life. It also allows us to observe what's going on in our body and mind in the present moment, as we respect the fact that our circumstances, feelings and needs are not static – especially in times of transition, such as during and after pregnancy. This kind of self-awareness allows us to truly know ourselves and thus truly nurture ourselves, which is why I am beginning the book here.

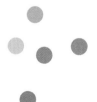

A note on values

Contentment is a universal pursuit. What brings us contentment, however, is unique to every person. To help you identify your values, reflect on your life experiences.

- When do you feel most happy?

- What behaviours, situations or interactions bring you personal satisfaction?

- When do you feel as though you are living the life you were born to live?

We hear a lot about what we should want, what we should do and what should make us happy, and this can distract us from what it is we actually want. As you tune in and reflect, be open to what you hear. Losing my older brother unexpectedly, when I was 22 years old, taught me how fleeting and fragile life is, and helped me to see with clarity how I wished to spend my days. That is, connecting with and nurturing others and savouring small, everyday joys.

After finishing my degree in nutrition and dietetics, I made some decisions that would allow me to live in line with my values. I lived frugally and moved to an area that had cheap rent so I could balance my days working as a dietitian – which I needed in order to earn money to live (and I do, thankfully, enjoy this work) – with days at home doing the things that brought me the most fulfilment: writing, cooking and being with those I love.

Grief had the same effect on Ben (my then boyfriend, now husband), who felt the loss of my brother deeply, having known him since he was 16. After reflecting on the things that brought him true satisfaction, Ben re-evaluated the decisions he had made up until that point simply because they seemed like the right thing to do, and made a career change.

In making these changes, Ben and I have both found ourselves to be more content. We're certainly not living in a perpetual state of happiness – that's not real life. But we do feel as though we are living a life of integrity – that is, one in line with our values.

Connecting to your inner self and having these discussions with your partner is a good idea before entering into parenthood. You may like to make a list itemising the things you both value most – kindness, achievement, respect, honesty, adventure, family, and so on. If your core values align, you will, no doubt, experience less conflict day to day. Regardless, an awareness of, and respect for, what drives you can help you to better support each other throughout this transition.

Be aware, though, that what drives us can change. While our core, fundamental values often remain the same throughout life, our perspective and desires can be altered (whether permanently or just for a season) based on our experiences – such as becoming a parent. Not every mother will experience a big or permanent shift in her values, but many do experience a dissonance between their pre-baby values and those of their new-mother self. Rather than assuming how you will feel once your baby arrives, try to be open, patient and flexible as you settle in to your new life.

How to tune in

Life is fast and full of distractions. In order to tune in, you need to pause and pay attention. Mindful practices are often at odds with our busy, overstimulated lives, and that is precisely why they're crucial. We need to get back in touch with how we are feeling, and not to attach judgement to what it is we uncover when tuning in.

Initially, it might feel strange to stop and listen, but soon enough it can become second nature. It's helpful to know that you may need to try a few different ways of connecting before you find a technique that resonates with you.

MINDFULNESS

One option to help you tune in is to engage in a mindful practice. The goal is mindfulness – that is, an awareness of yourself in the present moment. It can be brief or long – whatever feels good and is achievable.

If you can, find somewhere quiet and comfortable, whether outside in nature or indoors, such as a cosy chair or a warm bath. Don't worry if you can only find time when standing in a noisy, crowded train, though – mindfulness still works in these situations, and can be really useful to help you feel calm and centred. Wherever you are, bring your attention to your body and to your breathing. Notice how you are feeling and let go of any judgement that may arise when doing so. For example, 'I feel tired', 'The sun on my cheek feels warm', 'I feel restless'.

If thoughts enter your mind ('What should I make for dinner tonight?') or if you find yourself getting caught up in a critical, internal dialogue ('I feel so tired. Ugh, I shouldn't have stayed up late. Why do I do that to myself?!'), simply bring yourself back to your body and your breath – in and out, in and out. These intrusive thoughts are normal and commonly occur. It can be helpful to picture them as clouds in the sky, moving across your mind as you let them pass.

Mindfulness practice of this nature has been shown to have numerous benefits beyond self-awareness – it can strengthen our immune system and help in the management of depression, anxiety and stress. As we are more vulnerable to mental health issues during and after pregnancy, mindfulness can be extremely beneficial for pregnant women and new mothers. Even if you feel like you're not doing much by simply observing your thoughts and feelings, research confirms you are. Some days the practice will seem difficult and many thoughts will enter your mind, and that's ok. All that matters is you take the time to stop and pay attention without judgement.

MOVING

Our bodies are made to move. When we are active, we see great improvements in our physiological and psychological health. In our current, weight-obsessed culture, however, the word 'exercise' can have negative connotations. We tend to associate it with lacing up our sneakers and burning kilojoules as compensation for the food we ate when we were being 'naughty'. As a non-diet dietitian, this worries me.

I find the simple switch of calling exercise 'moving' helps to make it the positive, energising and enriching experience it should be. The type of movement for which our body yearns will change from season to season (and even day to day), so be sure to tune in to what feels good. And know that when you move – whether you're walking, stretching or dancing – you will feel happier, sleep better and be more connected to what is happening in your body and mind.

WRITING AND TALKING

The act of putting your thoughts and feelings on paper (or typing on a device) is incredibly beneficial to your mental health. Writing allows you to clear your mind of worrying thoughts, while giving you the opportunity to gain perspective over them. It can also help you to observe patterns between your feelings and the situations that may trigger them. You don't have to expend energy analysing what you've written in order for it to be valuable. In fact, sometimes you're better off just dumping whatever is in your brain onto the page, knowing you can throw it out once it's done.

If writing isn't appealing to you, consider talking. Verbally sharing your thoughts and feelings is similarly beneficial to writing, in that it allows you to express them. Suppressing or bottling up our emotions negatively affects our individual wellbeing and our relationships, whereas talking to a counsellor or confidant can help you to better understand yourself and your circumstances. It can also help you to adopt a more accepting and compassionate mindset towards yourself and others.

BARE FEET ON THE GROUND

When life feels chaotic (or even when it doesn't), one of my favourite ways to tune out the noise of the world and tune in to myself is to place my bare feet on the ground. Personally, I prefer grass, but sand works well, too (as does dirt, if you're fine with a bit of mess). 'Earthing', as this act is often called, has become a popular practice in recent years, as we begin to recognise the benefits of physically connecting with nature – something we don't do nearly enough in our modern world. I heartily encourage you to try it.

2, 2 AND 2

My mother taught me this final practice when I was a child. She would use it as a way of calming my nerves before ballet performances and school exams. Very simply, '2, 2 and 2' involves noticing two things in your environment you can smell, two things you can see and two things you can feel. If one of these doesn't appeal, you can replace it with two things you can hear.

Engaging with your senses in this manner forces you out of your head (and all its clutter and concerns) and back into your body in the present moment. What's great about this exercise is that it's particularly useful in situations where you are limited by time or physical space, such as when you're commuting or at your desk. Try it whenever you feel distracted, out of touch or overwhelmed with anxious thoughts.

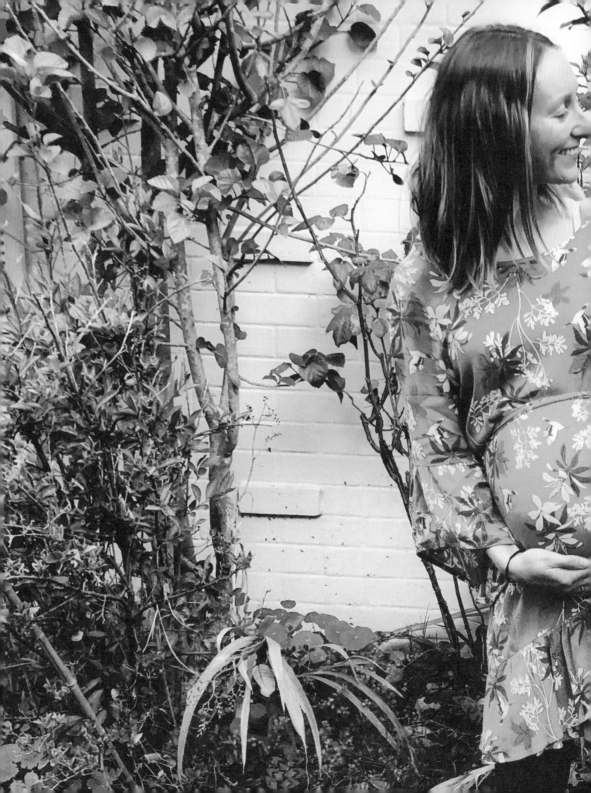

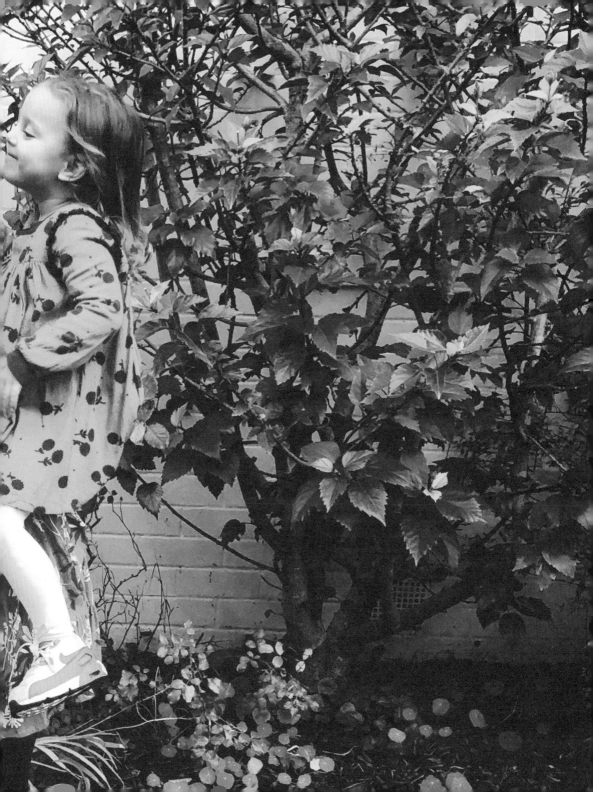

Ben favours a short, guided mindful meditation exercise. Every evening, he sits for 10 minutes and notices his breath and body while listening to an app on his phone. Sometimes he finishes the session feeling rejuvenated, and sometimes he continues to be distracted by thoughts. And sometimes he falls asleep.

Regardless of how he feels afterwards, Ben's mini-meditation practice, which he started after Joan was born as a means of managing work and life stress, is hugely beneficial. It allows him to strengthen the communication between his body and mind, affording him the opportunity to recognise his thoughts and feelings with clarity and compassion. As a result, he finds he can care for himself and communicate with others more effectively. We both notice when he gets out of his meditation habit (and I expect his employees may, too).

I prefer to tune in a little differently – by moving my body. Every morning when I get out of bed, and whenever I feel the need during the day, I take a moment to stretch and breathe. Before the birth of my second child, I would follow this practice with a walk outside, pushing Joan in her stroller while she ate a snack. Being in nature is a bonus and really amps up my mind–body connection.

My morning moving ritual gets good energy flowing, while connecting me to my body. This puts me in a state of awareness so that I can notice the signals my body is giving me, and tailor my self-care accordingly. That's one of the great benefits of mindfulness – the ability to identify what we need in order to feel well.

MY INNER VOICE

Here are some examples of the kinds of feelings I have discovered while stretching and moving, and my subsequent self-care response:

- 'You're tired ... go for a walk outside and eat your power foods – eggs and veggies – for breakfast. Fresh air is just as energising as the ten cups of coffee you're craving and, unlike the coffee, it'll give you long-lasting energy to make it through the day.'

- 'You're unsettled ... something doesn't feel right. Perhaps it's because you got hardly any work done yesterday. Joan is now napping only once a day, and you're lucky if it lasts an hour (who are these children who nap for 2–3 hours?!). It's time to create a more structured work time. Brainstorm a few ideas and talk to Ben on the weekend about where to go from here.'

- 'You're anxious ... it's understandable: you just found out your friend is pregnant and you're worried that after your miscarriage you won't get pregnant for a long time. Trust your body, be patient and go eat some cake.'

The recognition and response don't always happen with the click of my fingers as the above dialogue suggests, but while I'm moving through the meditative motions of stretching or walking, my thoughts clear and I am free to sense what I am feeling and what I am needing. Studies show a positive correlation between mindfulness and self-compassion, suggesting that when we tune in we are, in fact, compelled to treat ourselves in a beneficial way by honouring the needs of both our present and future selves.

Tuning in during pregnancy and beyond

Every day, women become mothers. The transition to motherhood itself is not unique, but our individual experience of it is. From whether you had an uncomplicated pregnancy, to the nature of your baby's birth, to your health postnatally, there is nothing cookie-cutter about creating a family. Indeed, there are endless ways for your experience to differ from that of other mothers. That is why we need to tune in and pay attention to what is going on in our little world as we go through this universal yet very personal process of becoming a mother.

Try connecting to your body and baby during pregnancy by practising the mindfulness exercise described on pages 14–15. Tune in to how you feel overall – note, for example, whether you feel peaceful or anxious, sore or comfortable. Then draw your attention to your belly and your baby. As you breathe, notice any sensations you are feeling within your body in relation to your baby. Take note of the way your belly feels (hard, soft, itchy, large); any movements you notice; and the overall energy you feel coming from within.

Mindful practices during pregnancy can help you to feel grounded throughout all the changes you are experiencing, and connect you to the little person (or people) you are growing. The practices can also help you to recognise when something feels off. Maternal intuition is something to respect and cultivate – obstetricians and midwives always

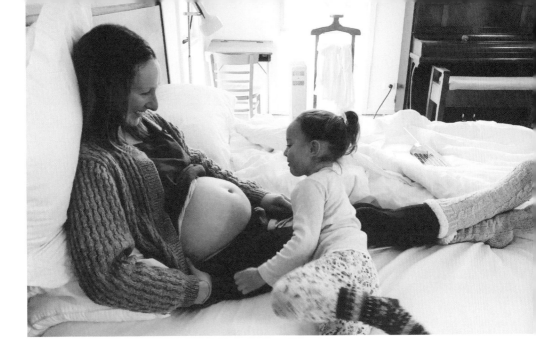

encourage mothers to verbalise when something doesn't seem right, whether it concerns their baby's health or their own. You can do the same mindfulness exercise after pregnancy, too, by allowing yourself to first connect to yourself and then your baby. Again, this will help you to figure out more easily when something feels right or wrong, as well as the type of self-care and support you may be needing. You may not notice much at all, and that's fine – remember, you're strengthening your mind–body connection just by paying attention. Try tuning in when you're both at peace (such as while your baby is napping or feeding), and simply breathe and notice, breathe and notice.

Connecting to ourselves and to our baby in this manner was arguably easier to do before we became so electronically connected to others and easily distracted. These days, with just the click of a button we have instant access to a world of information – and misinformation! – through online articles and forums, and the countless pregnancy and parenting books we can buy or borrow. As a result, it has become almost a reflex to look outside of ourselves for answers.

At the same time, we are constantly seeing curated snapshots of other people's lives (via social media and the media in general), and this makes it harder for us to both tune in to our world, and feel content with our unfiltered reality. Images of pregnant women sipping green juice wearing cute, bump-hugging outfits, and pictures of babies sleeping soundly in their cots can lead even the most level-headed woman to feel discontented.

I am not suggesting we disconnect completely. Social media has given us the ability to meet people from all over the world, most of whom we otherwise wouldn't have known, and these connections can be immensely valuable (for example, if you're going through a particular experience to which people in your inner circle or community cannot relate). In addition, the internet has provided us with videos on topics like how to use baby carriers and wraps, as well as access to books and apps on things like infant brain development – all of which can positively influence our parenting experience. But we do need to be intentional about what and who we are connecting to.

To maintain your positive sense of self during pregnancy and motherhood, strive to do the following:

- Unfollow or block social media accounts that make you feel ashamed, discontented or just plain bad.

- Remember that everyone has their challenging moments, they are simply not shared as often as the #blessed ones.

- In real life and online, surround yourself with those who speak honestly about all facets of the parenthood experience, who inspire you to feel gratitude for what you have and who empower you to trust your ability as a mother.

- Remember the importance of context. By this I mean who you are, who your baby is, who your partner is (if you have one), each of your physical and mental health needs, who your support network is, what your home situation is like, if you are working in addition to mothering, what hours you and/or your partner work, and so on. All of this information is highly individual and relevant when making decisions about your baby's care, as well as your own.

- Whenever possible, seek personalised advice from a professional who can consider your context and give informed advice. This is especially important for issues that are making you feel worried or concerned, because searching for answers online may cause you additional stress. If the advice you receive doesn't sit well, get a second opinion.

- Pay attention to your body and baby. You may not have a degree in childhood development or medicine, but you are the expert on your family – with insights no-one else can possibly have.

Cultivating gratitude

Life is multicoloured. There are moments of brightness and joy, and moments of darkness and suffering. We all, at times, experience challenges and feel discontent – even when living a life that is in line with our values and following our intuition. When this happens (and as we wait for events to transpire, decisions to be made or time to pass), we need to nurture ourselves with extra tenderness. Taking note of what you are thankful for can help summon positive feelings when it feels as though you don't have much to be grateful for.

Let me pause and create an impromptu gratitude list of my own. Right now, I am grateful for:

- the three peaceful, uninterrupted hours I have to write while my husband is with our children

- the gentle morning light dancing on my desk

- the coffee I made this morning, which tastes more delicious than usual and (joy, oh joy) is still hot

- my parents – in general, but specifically for the dinner they brought over last night. And for the fact that they obliged my family's early-bird preference so we could get to bed early after a wakeful night. Did I mention I'm grateful for coffee?

- my health, the health of my loved ones, and the fact that we are here to live this day together.

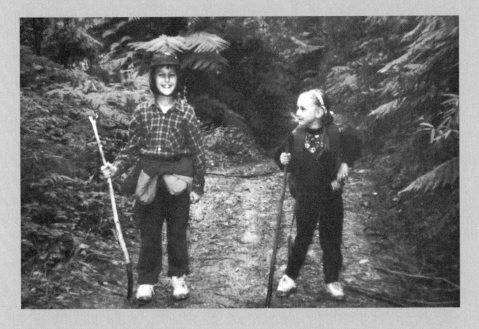

That last one is my personal mic drop. You know when a person is speaking on a stage and they say something so powerful and perfect that they drop their microphone and walk away because positively nothing more needs to be said? That's how I feel about the final note on my list – it instantly summons deep gratitude that I am here at all. The loss of my brother taught me how, in an instant, that can change. And what I take from his loss is the ability to filter through what matters at the end of the day and what doesn't.

We all need a little nudge towards positivity and acceptance every now and then, and studies show a gratitude practice, like this one, can be immensely effective in achieving optimism and improving our overall wellbeing. Even when life is peachy, it serves us to reflect on the little and big things we are grateful for.

Intuition

As soon as I found out I was pregnant the first time, I felt certain I was having a girl. Not too long after that, I changed my mind. He was a boy. Yep, I knew I was having a boy. Ben and I had both wanted to wait until the birth to find out whether we were having a boy or a girl, and although I didn't mind either way, I spent a lot of time wondering.

All the prediction tricks contradicted each other. When I was noticeably pregnant, a woman at the grocery store proclaimed, 'Girls take your beauty!' before promptly telling me she believed I was having a girl. Another lady asked me to turn around so she could observe my buttocks – apparently the shape of my backside meant my baby was a boy. As it turns out, my bottom was misleading. Or, more accurately, old wives' tales are misleading (and, sometimes, rather insulting).

No matter your baby's heart rate, what foods you're craving or how you're carrying, unless you opt to find out, there is no way to know the sex of your baby before you meet them at birth. And while some profess a strong intuition about the matter, we cannot rely on it to tell us this information, either. But that's ok, because our intuition serves an entirely different purpose – that is, to help guide us through life.

You might like to think of your intuition as your internal guiding light – illuminating insights without conscious and analytical thought. The concept of intuition and how we develop this instinctive knowledge about something or someone is still poorly understood by science, though research suggests that intuitive insights are informed by our past experiences, as well as our perception of the world around us. It should be noted, then, that individuals who have experienced trauma or abuse may have skewed perceptions as a result of their traumatic past experiences. You might like to reflect on whether following your intuition has historically led you to positive outcomes, as it ideally should. If it hasn't, you may want to seek support from a psychologist. Generally speaking, though, there is value to be gained from listening to our intuition. Especially when we become mothers.

Mothers are said to develop a maternal intuition in order to help them care for their baby, who is born highly dependent, immature and in need of nurturing. Yet because a person's intuition draws upon their past experiences, when it comes to first-time mothers, that maternal intuition will also be immature and in need of nurturing. Even if you have looked after babies in the past, caring for your own, with your hormonally charged, postnatal body, is an entirely different experience.

So how do we help our maternal intuition to grow? As stated earlier, making time to tune in regularly will help put you in a state of awareness, whereby you're more likely to recognise any intuitive insights.

The other thing you can do is give it time. Allow yourself to gain experiences – both positive and negative ones. Take your baby's cries, for example. Mothers are said to know intuitively what their baby needs upon hearing them cry, but this sense of knowing can take a little while to develop. For me, it was a case of trial and error before I instinctively knew what my first baby needed. And even then, I didn't get it right every time, as I was sleep deprived or second-guessing myself after getting lost in a vortex of online advice, much of which is incorrect.

Know that when you struggle and make mistakes, it's all information to be filed away to inform the intuitive messages your future self will receive.

AN EXERCISE TO ACCESS YOUR INTUITION

If you're unsure what it feels like to receive an intuitive message, try the following exercise.

- Find a situation where you have a variety of options. It could be as trivial as ordering from a menu or something more significant, like selecting a health care provider during pregnancy or a daycare centre for your baby. Whatever the situation, notice how you feel when you lean one way versus another.

- As a way of deciding, you could flip a coin – if it lands on heads, go with option A; if it lands on tails, go with option B. When the coin comes down, notice whether you feel disappointed or relieved by the outcome. If you are relieved, that's a sign that that particular option was the right choice for you.

- Reflect on possible ways your body was trying to tell you this before the coin toss. Did you have a gut feeling? For me, when something goes against my intuition, I register a sensation of unease in my chest. Conversely, when something feels right, I notice a rush of calm energy move across my body.

Even if it's a scary or challenging prospect, I feel energised and affirmed when considering the path that is in line with my intuition, and one could argue that this is because intuitive messages seek to move us towards people and situations that serve us and away from those that don't. It's this energised and affirmed feeling that I seek when making decisions as a mother – be it about my baby's sleep needs or whether my toddler needs a day of rest at home. Finally, it's important to note that sometimes there isn't a clear 'right' answer; one option may just feel better than the other.

USING ADVICE TO AFFIRM YOUR INTUITION

New parents invariably receive an influx of unsolicited advice about how to care for their baby and themselves – from sources as varied as family members and strangers at the supermarket. And while these instructions tend to come from a loving place and can even be helpful, it's easy for new mothers to feel overwhelmed and sensitive, wishing everyone would just mind their own business.

Why not use it to your advantage? If the advice you have been offered is relevant, and has been delivered respectfully, it may help you affirm your intuition. Whether or not you follow their advice doesn't matter, as simply pondering their suggestion may help clarify what feels right to you. If doing so makes you feel frazzled, or if you find your mind too cluttered with other people's opinions to recognise what feels right to you, go ahead and stop the conversation. Importantly, set boundaries that protect your mental wellbeing. You may find, however, that by considering their opinion, you end up more confident in yours.

Gut feeling

When someone reflects on a time when they knew something was true or right, they often say they had a 'gut feeling' about it. This makes sense, as the gut is often referred to as our 'second brain'. Located within our stomach, and along the entire gastrointestinal tract, is our enteric nervous system (ENS) – which houses millions of neurons that communicate with the brain and influence its actions.

When confronted with a situation that is perceived as stressful, a number of instinctive, protective responses are triggered within the body, giving you a 'gut feeling' that something is wrong. Many individuals register a similar feeling when they access their intuition.

In recent years, research has given us a greater understanding of, and appreciation for, our gut and its role in health. We now know that the gut has the ability to produce hormones and other substances that influence our appetite, digestion (nutrient absorption happens in the gut), immunity, mood, mental health and overall wellbeing. We also know that certain environments (excess stress, for example) can alter our bacterial and hormonal balance in a way that negatively impacts our appetite, mood, and so on.

It therefore benefits us to pay attention to any gut feelings we might have – not just in terms of our intuition, but how well we feel in our body – and to take care of this powerful system with supportive dietary and lifestyle practices.

Regularly tuning in is a good place to start, as it will allow you to notice sensations that arise which could be related to digestion, stress or both. Indeed, stress and gut health are inextricably linked, and any endeavour to vitalise our gut should involve stress and anxiety management.

Getting adequate sleep is also greatly important, as is our food intake. Foods rich in fibre are supportive of good gut health – specifically prebiotics, which are found in some vegetables, fruits and wholegrains such as raw oats (to name just a few foods).

If you have an intolerance to certain foods, such as dairy or gluten, your gut will be happier when you avoid them. Be sure, however, to not restrict your diet too much, as a varied diet is necessary for a healthy gut.

Finally, foods or supplements that are rich in probiotics (that is, beneficial bacteria) can be helpful, especially after taking antibiotics. Probiotic-rich foods include fermented vegetables (such as sauerkraut and kimchi), kefir and yoghurt with live cultures. It's important to note that not all probiotic supplements are created equal, so it's a good idea to seek guidance from a dietitian when deciding what is right for you.

For personalised advice on gut health, I encourage you to make an appointment with a holistically minded dietitian, as well as a mental health professional, to help you manage any feelings of stress and anxiety.

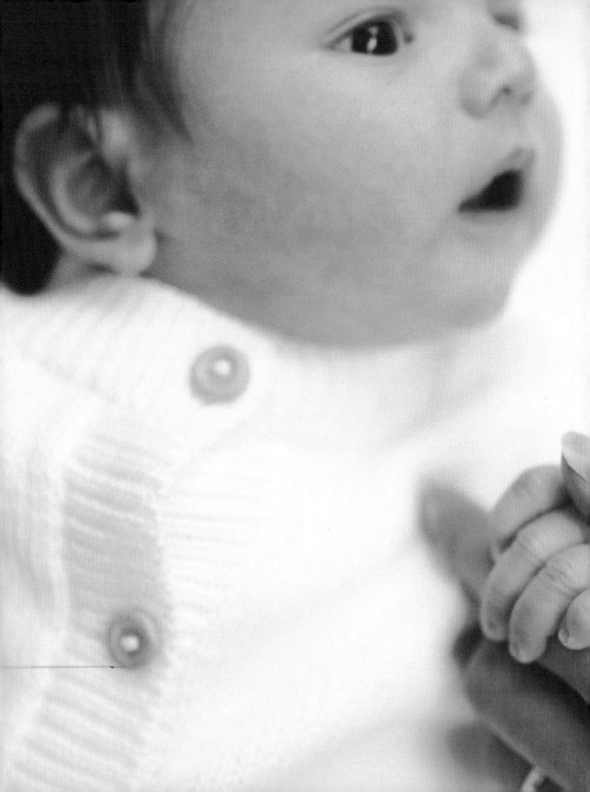

Chapter 2
Expectations and Compassion

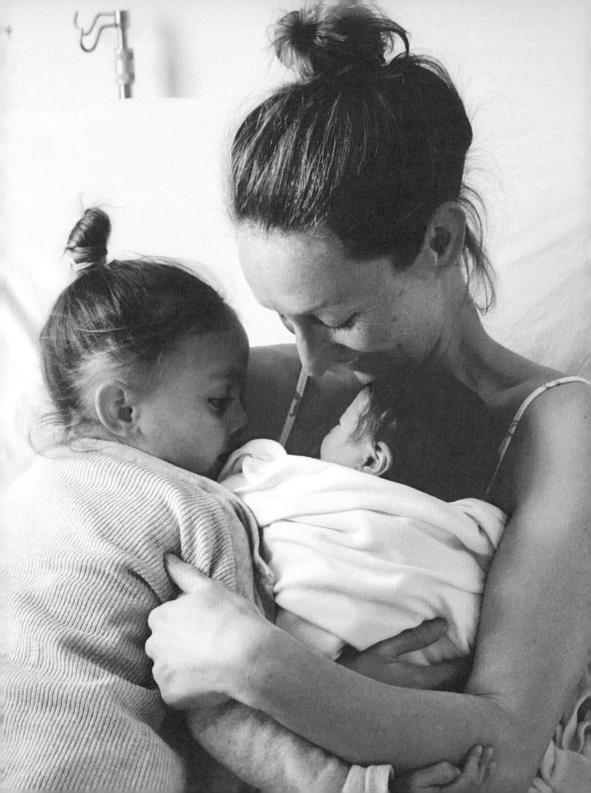

In our present culture, there is a tremendous gap between the idealised version of pregnancy and motherhood, and the reality. That is not to say real life is unpleasant. When you become a mother you may experience more joy and fulfilment than ever before. But you may also find your new life is different from what you expected.

There is a duality to the experience, as many of the beautiful moments coexist with the hard ones. We hear our baby's first laugh while dealing with a bout of mastitis; we see them take their first steps while feeling completely shattered with exhaustion; we hear them tell their first joke while lying on the couch recovering from a miscarriage. That is the nature of motherhood – and life in general – but it's not necessarily what we expect.

Recent studies on maternal health have shown that parents-to-be require better education about normal infant behaviour and postnatal realities, so that they can have more realistic expectations of both their babies and themselves. Essentially, we need our jaws to drop a little less (we also need support systems in place, which I'll discuss further in Chapter 3: Support), because when we are open to having a motley experience that is tremendously joyful and tremendously challenging, we can more easily accept the challenges and make ourselves available to the joy.

I had my own expectations about what life with a newborn would be like. And while expectations are not always false or damaging, they do become problematic when we rigidly hold onto them in the face of a deviating reality (the fact that our expectations tend to be based on an idealised version of what we hope for means this can often happen).

Take Joan's sleep behaviour, for example. Despite my efforts to encourage an independent sleeper (trust me, I tried all the gentle tricks and I did them well), she insisted on remaining close to me. Her preference came as a shock to Ben and me, who thought a tired baby would just sleep – end of story. As a new mother, I had internalised the rhetoric that there is a specific formula parents need to follow in order to have a 'good' baby who will sleep through the night and away from their mother. I didn't yet know that while these recommendations work for many babies, some simply have different natures and needs. With all the talk about creating bad sleep habits running through my brain, I would hold my sleeping daughter in my arms and feel like a failure. I felt like a failure for responding to her needs – how nuts is that?

It was only when I better educated myself about newborn sleeping behaviour (see more in Chapter 5: Sleep) and accepted Joan's disposition, that I was able to find contentment in my circumstances. Her needs didn't change but my expectations did, and we were both happier.

No doubt we will all experience our expectations being shattered at some point along our motherhood journey. This can happen before we even hold our baby, such as in the case of fertility issues, miscarriage, and pregnancy or birth complications. As a pre- and postnatal dietitian, I counsel many women who, soon after their positive pregnancy test, are incapable of nourishing themselves and their growing baby in their ideal way, due to the onset of food aversions and nausea. Many cite this as their first experience of 'mummy guilt' – possibly even 'mummy shame' – and it is our propensity to feel these emotions that we must first address.

Guilt versus shame

For the initial 18 weeks of my first pregnancy, I couldn't eat vegetables without gagging. On the other hand, the very thought of a fast-food burger would appease my nausea. I found it all incredibly bizarre and wrote about it on my blog. To this day, that post has generated the greatest number of emails from readers located all over the world – far more than anything else I have written. These emails all begin similarly, along the lines of, 'Thank you so much for sharing your experience of first-trimester sickness. I have been feeling incredibly guilty for not being able to eat how I usually do.' It's not uncommon for women who previously enjoyed a variety of vibrant, flavourful foods to want nothing more than plain toast or potatoes in the early weeks of pregnancy. For most, this change is temporary, kicking in around week 6 and lasting until week 12, give or take a few weeks. In the scheme of things that's not a long time, but it's long enough for lots of women to experience a hearty dose of mummy guilt.

Generally speaking – and in psychological terms – guilt refers to the feeling you get when you've done something you know or believe to be bad or wrong, and your concern for the negative impact it may have on yourself or another person. It's not a particularly nice thing to experience and yet, interestingly, feeling guilty isn't necessarily a bad thing. In small doses, and in situations where this feeling is warranted (like when you have done something that is either wrong or goes against your values), guilt can act as a type of moral compass – offering us the chance to change our behaviour or make amends with whomever we believe we have hurt.

Shame refers to a person feeling bad about themselves, believing that they, not their behaviours, are fundamentally bad. Unlike guilt, which can be useful, shame can be an insidious emotion that may lead to self-loathing, isolation (in an attempt to shield ourselves from experiencing it again), and feelings of anger, anxiety, helplessness and worthlessness. Shame has the potential to be really harmful and, unfortunately, it's an easy emotion to feel.

In our present culture, where we are constantly inundated with conflicting messages about the 'right' way to feed ourselves, it's almost impossible not to experience negative feelings in relation to food. Everyone seems to have an opinion on the matter, and many share their opinions passionately (often forcefully) in the hope that others will eat as they do, without necessarily appreciating the fact that what works for one person or body, won't always work for another. You see, there is no one diet or way of eating that will universally satisfy all our needs.

While I enjoy eating bread made from wheat, my friend with coeliac disease cannot have one crumb without harming her health. Similarly, another friend favours eggs for breakfast, yet she cannot feed them to her daughter, who has an egg allergy. My father generally feels better eating fewer carbohydrate-rich foods than my mother does, despite the fact that he is taller and larger. And then there's my cousin, who likes pineapple on her pizza, whereas I prefer a margherita.

Research does suggest that certain foods are likely to benefit most individuals – such as vegetables, legumes, fruit, nuts, seeds, oily fish and extra-virgin olive oil – but no two bodies are the same. And what's more, our needs and preferences change as we move through life. The only way to know what works for you in your present season is to stop focusing on rules or fads and to tune in to your own body. Then, instead of feeling guilty for not doing as your friend does, or for eating food other people tell you is 'bad', you can save your guilt for the times you find yourself consistently making choices that don't serve you and your needs, and allow it to encourage you to be a little more mindful of your food intake – whatever that looks like.

Note: If you're struggling to identify the types of foods that make you feel good, that your body thrives on and that you enjoy eating, or if you're struggling to give yourself permission to eat these foods (all of which is highly understandable given our current food culture), I encourage you to seek the guidance of a dietitian who is also a certified Intuitive Eating counsellor, or one familiar with the non-diet approach (see page 310 for some helpful resources).

We all want to be the best mothers we can, and give our growing baby all it needs to thrive. So I appreciate why some women feel guilty for not eating their best during pregnancy. The thing is, most don't need to feel quite as guilty as they do. The reason you may not be loading your plate with vegetables could be that veggies, and food in general, can either make you feel like vomiting or actually cause you to vomit. You're gravitating towards plain toast for a reason. And do you know what? In the long run, a temporary break from broccoli, or another food that's causing unpleasant symptoms, will be fine.

While it's undoubtedly beneficial for both you and your baby to eat a nutritious and balanced diet during pregnancy (more in chapters 6 and 7), the period of time in which your plate looks more beige than green is brief. If you have eaten a varied diet full of nutrient-rich foods in the months and years leading up to the onset of pregnancy sickness, you will have created a healthy foundation from which your baby can draw nourishment and gain the nutrients they require. On top of this, a quality prenatal supplement taken as directed will help cover your nutritional needs.

Of course, some women struggle with nausea well into their second trimester, and others for their entire pregnancy, so it's important to consider your unique situation and seek medical advice to ensure you're

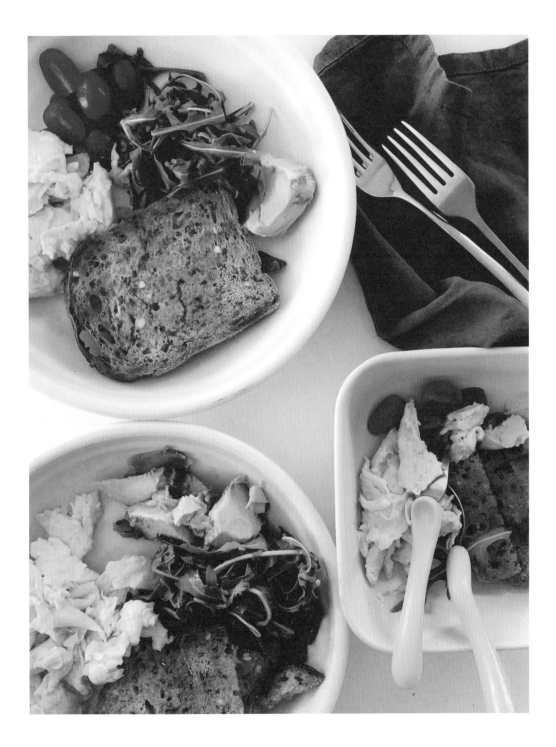

able to nourish yourself. Most women, however, do experience some relief – whether the sickness gradually subsides on its own, becomes tolerable with a few tricks (such as those listed on pages 200–5) or with the use of anti-nausea medication prescribed by your health care provider. On the challenging days, remember that it is better to eat and drink something rather than nothing. And if you're consistently struggling to keep down any foods and fluids, seek medical assistance immediately to avoid dehydration.

Now if your eating habits before conception weren't all that great, you can leverage any guilt you may be feeling to nudge yourself towards more nourishing practices that will benefit both you and your baby. That's the beauty of guilt; when we recognise the emotion without judging or scolding ourselves for our behaviour, we can use it to our advantage.

Say you found yourself doing something that went against your values (for me, that might be yelling at my children or husband). Any guilt you may feel can propel you to apologise, identify why this particular guilt-inducing behaviour may have happened and encourage you to put systems in place so that you're less likely to do it in the future.

Of course, we can't always remedy our guilt so easily. Sometimes we will wrestle with this emotion for longer than we'd like; and sometimes reality means we are unable to act in accordance with our values, so our guilt will hang around. For example, if nausea persists for all 9 months despite medical intervention, if we cannot breastfeed despite wanting to or if we must return to work earlier than we wish. Perhaps that is why mummy guilt is so often discussed – because real life means we can't always parent in our ideal way, especially when women are expected to do and be everything without the necessary support. In these instances, we need to be kind to ourselves, and perhaps say the Serenity Prayer: '… Grant me the serenity to accept the things I cannot change, the courage to change the things I can, and the wisdom to know the difference.'

If all of this sounds completely absurd to you, if you cannot fathom ever feeling ok about your 'bad' behaviour or accept acting against your values, it's possible that you're experiencing not just guilt but shame.

When our sense of self is challenged, and when we feel embarrassed, judged or as though we have done something wrong, we open ourselves up to shame and all its negative flow-on effects. 'Mummy shame' (that is, a woman believing she is a bad mother) can hit us at any point on our motherhood journey, though we are particularly vulnerable when entering the postnatal period as first-time mothers, when so much of what we experience is new. In this season, we are given endless opportunities to question and compare our actions and abilities. We may also be feeling flat and isolated – conditions that help shame to thrive.

It's crucial, then, that we nurture our new-mother selves and build up resilience to the shame-inducing voices (whether inside our head or from other people) that directly or inadvertently say, 'You're not good enough.' If we hear that critical dialogue often enough, we can start to believe it.

Acceptance and compassion

How do we manage our guilt and build resilience to shame? First, we need to recognise what it is we are feeling. If this sort of self-awareness doesn't come easily to you, you may wish to set aside a specific time each day to pay attention to what is going on in your body and mind (such as before you get out of bed in the morning, while you are in the shower or when your baby is napping). Doing so will help you to create a habit of listening, which will ultimately allow awareness to come to you more easily as you go about your life.

Once you have acknowledged your feelings, the next step is to offer yourself acceptance and compassion for any undesirable ones, as well as the behaviours or events that brought them on. Say we are berating ourselves for a decision we made about our baby's care that we now regret. Acceptance and compassion will allow us to move past the mistakes we make and help us to remain confident in our role as our baby's carer. Research tells us our ability to do this – that is, to compassionately accept ourselves – is a strong predictor of an individual's happiness. That's because acceptance moves us away from thoughts such as 'Why me?' to thoughts like 'What now?' while compassion moves us from thoughts such as 'I'm a failure' to thoughts like 'I'm human.'

After all, no-one is perfect or has a perfect life – we all experience difficulties and make mistakes. A compassionate and accepting mindset helps us come out the other end of life's challenges with an intact, and possibly even strengthened, sense of self. Most people don't treat themselves in this manner, though. When we fail to live up to our ideals or things don't go as planned, our cultural tendency is to compare and criticise.

Dr Kristin Neff, a self-compassion researcher, demonstrates the value of offering ourselves compassion in these instances. She describes compassion as 'a kind, connected, and clear-sighted way of relating to ourselves', which can help us to better manage our negative emotions and experiences so that we don't overidentify with them. This means we are less likely to end up dwelling, catastrophising (believing the situation worse than it is), internalising (allowing it to become part of our identity) and getting lost in a shame spiral. Acceptance plus compassion is a formidable combination, one that will serve you well throughout motherhood, and life in general.

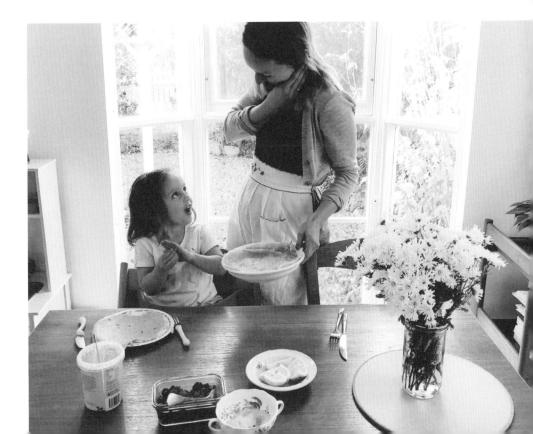

- Repeat the following mantra: 'I'm human. Nobody is perfect, we all make mistakes and we all experience challenges. I'm feeling challenged right now.'

- Ask yourself how you would treat a friend in your situation. What advice would you give them?

- Talk to someone about how you are feeling. Verbalising your thoughts allows you to gain perspective on them.

- Do something nurturing for yourself, such as making yourself a cup of tea, taking a warm bath or going for a walk.

- Try one or more of the tuning-in exercises listed on pages 14–17, with the goal of noticing how you are feeling without judgement. The more we do this, the easier it becomes to bring in acceptance and compassion.

- Try a gratitude practice, such as the one described on pages 26–7.

If you are unable to do this nifty brain work on your own, don't worry. Many people struggle to recognise what it is they are feeling, let alone give themselves acceptance and compassion. If you feel you need help, I encourage you to seek the guidance of a psychologist. This is especially important if you're dealing with trauma or mental health issues, as you may require support when working through your feelings.

A note on self-worth

It's pertinent to note that it's easier to reject shame and receive acceptance and compassion if we believe we are worthy of acceptance and compassion. That is, if we have a strong sense of self-worth. The way we are raised plays a role in the development of this belief. If, as children, we felt unconditionally loved, if we were encouraged to try, and if we were accepted and supported when we failed, we are more likely to have a strong sense of self-worth. This means we are more likely to be more optimistic and more able to treat ourselves with kindness as we experience the ups and downs of life. It doesn't all come down to our childhood – the experience of trauma or shame can challenge our self-worth at any age. Nevertheless, the early childhood years are crucial for brain development, laying the groundwork for the way we process and react to our life experiences.

If you wish to strengthen your sense of self-worth, psychologists and researchers have identified mindfulness to be a particularly effective method. Essentially, it rewires your brain in such a way that it becomes easier to be positive and give yourself, and others, compassion. There are numerous other activities you can do to encourage this mindset – including asking a friend to list things they value in you (in the hope that you begin to see yourself as they do), and helping others who are in need of support. But there is something particularly attractive about the practice of tuning in mindfully, because the more you do it, the more instinctive it becomes.

Acceptance and compassion in relation to food and bodies

Now we'll explore the example of a woman who is experiencing a drastic change to her eating habits during early pregnancy. Let's call her Sarah. Say that Sarah wants nothing more at this time than toast and potato chips, and is feeling bad because of it. Shaming herself – by comparing her food intake with what she imagined pre-pregnancy or what her pregnant friends are eating – and labelling herself a bad mother is entirely unproductive.

Having a shame-filled mindset won't help Sarah eat in a 'better' way; what it will do is leave her vulnerable to feelings of stress, inadequacy and hopelessness. It also leaves her far more likely to overeat the foods she is shaming herself for wanting in the first place. If, on the other hand, Sarah were to find a way to tune in to how she was feeling, acknowledge and accept what was happening and treat herself with kindness, she would be better able to manage her toast and potato reality. She may still not be pleased that the range of food that presently appeals is limited, but she wouldn't waste her energy chastising herself for it.

Instead, she could pick herself up and figure out a way to best nourish herself in her current situation. This may be identifying her nausea triggers in order to reduce her symptoms, and/or seeking assistance from qualified health practitioners to help her through this challenging time. Sarah may also decide to ask her loved ones to assemble some meals, as food preparation can be one of the biggest roadblocks to nourishment at this time.

As you can see, acceptance and compassion lead to better outcomes by allowing you to free your mind of unproductive thoughts and think clearly. Essentially, it helps you treat yourself as you would a friend. In fact, that is precisely what Dr Neff recommends you do in order to become familiar with the act of giving yourself compassion.

Consider how you might treat a friend who is in your situation:

- Would you speak to a friend, especially one who was going through a challenging time, in a rude or severe manner? No.

- Would you tell a friend to suck it up, that other people were able to handle pregnancy so they should too? No.

- Would you tell them that their eating habits were disgusting and that from this point on they must only eat 'clean'? No.

And yet this is how many women (pregnant or not) speak to themselves when they fail to live up to their ideals, no matter how unrealistic they are.

- Additionally, would you tell a friend to forget about nutrition altogether? No, because doing so won't benefit your friend or her baby.

Self-compassion isn't about coddling. Rather, it assists you, through level-headed kindness, in making the best possible choice in your given circumstances. It helps you to see that you are worthy of kindness and care even when you fall short of your ideals, which is revolutionary, really, when you consider the way our culture trains us to think harshly of our bodies and eating habits, and to compare and criticise ourselves.

Food, bodies and shame

As a dietitian, I have counselled people of all ages and genders, and from all socioeconomic backgrounds, through feelings of shame surrounding their food intake and body size/shape. We live in a culture that praises one body type (thin) and denigrates everything else, based on the hazardous assumption that thinness equals health and beauty, and fatness equals the opposite.

The Health at Every Size and Body Positive movements are working to smash down diet culture and reduce body-size stigma. But we still have a long way to go, as people continue to make assumptions about a person's health and their behaviours based on their size, and provoke shame in order to promote weight loss – believing that doing so will lead to better health. Which it doesn't.

Shame can leave people feeling unimportant and unmotivated. It damages their self-esteem and leads them into destructive – not healthy – behaviours. In fact, research shows that shame is more closely correlated with eating disorders and depression than with health and happiness. We also know that diets don't work: they dysregulate a person's metabolism, so weight loss is rarely sustained after ceasing the restrictive behaviour that helped them to reduce their size. In most cases, people end up heavier and more discontent than they were before they started dieting.

Research has shown, however, that body acceptance and intuitive eating lead to eating behaviours that are supportive of good health, as well as improved psychological wellbeing. And yet we continue to speak critically of our bodies (our own and other peoples') and engage in yo-yo dieting – starting one restrictive, punishing diet and exercise regime, then rebelling against it before starting another. These behaviours negatively impact everyone, even our children.

From a heartbreakingly young age, we sense that our value as an individual lies in how closely we fit our culture's narrow description of beauty. We learn, by observing messages in the media and the behaviours of those close to us, to restrict whatever foods our culture is presently deeming 'bad' in order to reach or maintain a certain size. Thus, what we eat and how much we weigh become inextricably linked to our self-worth. Is it any wonder, then, that we feel shame when we find ourselves craving foods we've been told are naughty or dangerous, that we feel shame when our bodies grow and remain larger than they were before – whether during puberty, pregnancy, motherhood or menopause?

To help people move away from feelings of shame, which can inhibit their ability to properly nourish themselves, I try to get them to accept where they're at in the present moment. This doesn't mean they must start loving every inch of their body – that's not always realistic, certainly not if someone has spent years loathing and resisting the way they look. I do, however, challenge them to treat themselves as though they are in a place they already deem acceptable, in the hope of shifting their views of food (and themselves) to a more productive and nurturing place.

For many individuals, this sort of self-acceptance and compassion doesn't come easily. When it comes to food and our bodies, we're so used to restricting and reprimanding ourselves that bringing trust and kindness into the equation can feel scary. But this mindset doesn't, as some may fear, lead to apathy or reckless indulgence. What it actually leads to is increased motivation to engage in beneficial behaviours that are respectful and sustainable. This is because people who are self-compassionate have their best interests at heart, meaning they take into consideration their immediate needs, while also considering how any decisions they make will impact their wellbeing in the future.

This may look like resting your body at times and moving it at other times (instead of exercising out of punishment for what you ate, or to achieve a certain body shape or size). Essentially, it helps you to tune in and trust your body to tell you what it needs without the distracting influence of diet culture.

As you can see, it is infinitely more advantageous to our health to be accepting and kind. Though we won't be the only ones who benefit. Our children will too, as the way we care for, and relate to, ourselves will influence how they care for, and relate to, themselves. Even if it feels difficult to treat yourself and your body with compassion, do try. And know that in doing so, you will be showing your children that all bodies are deserving of love, care and respect, and this will help bolster their sense of self, as well as your own.

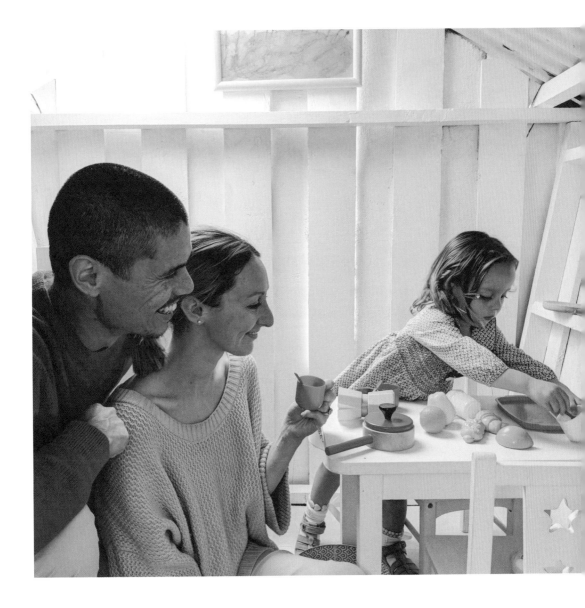

Let me give you one final nudge towards this style of thinking. Some women find it easier to be accepting and compassionate when they consider the profound physiological changes that occur in a woman's body when she becomes a mother. The fact that we grow an entire human and produce milk that is uniquely tailored to their needs, is a mic-drop statement in itself.

Of additional note are the neurological changes we experience. As Professor Laura Glynn explains, 'Pregnancy primes the brain for dramatic neuroplasticity, which is further stimulated by delivery, lactation and mother-child interactions.' Essentially, our brain changes its activities in order to facilitate mother–baby bonding and ensure we are attuned to our baby's needs. Our ability to do this – to alter our brains so that we can better care for our infants – is astounding. As is the fact that we can regulate our baby's temperature, heartbeat and breathing simply by holding them.

Research affirms just how awesome women's bodies are, which is pleasing for a number of reasons: first, it makes me feel like a goddess; secondly, it encourages self-acceptance and self-compassion when we are unable to 'bounce back' 2 weeks after giving birth (in fact, it makes it easier for us to call bullshit on that entire concept); and thirdly, by examining the changes women experience during and after pregnancy, we can better understand and support this transition on a societal level. Widespread ignorance propagates widespread unrealistic expectations, the outcome of which is a lack of support and respect for women as they go through matresence. This affects not only the wellbeing of the mother, but that of her baby and partner too. It affects us all.

Very few of our motherhood experiences will happen precisely as we'd hoped. As a mother, there are countless things I didn't expect or desire to happen, yet have had to accept. My inability to eat vegetables in early pregnancy and Joan's needs surrounding sleep are just two examples. Another is her hip dysplasia, which was diagnosed soon after her birth and required her to wear a brace essentially 24/7 for the first 3 months of her life. And then there are the two pregnancy losses Ben and I experienced between our first and second children. When these things happened we were devastated, of course (and I imagine I'll always carry the scars of my miscarriages); but when the initial shock wore off it felt so much better to be ok with it all. Acceptance doesn't mean rolling over and giving in, and it doesn't mean we must like every aspect of our reality. Rather, it helps us to feel ok when things are hard or simply different from what we imagined.

So, readers, why don't we let our expectations of new motherhood simply and boldly be this: that as we enter into this unfamiliar, dynamic and demanding season, we will be open to how our experience will unfold, and strive to treat ourselves with kindness. Let's remember that we need to give ourselves compassion just as much as we give it to our children. So that when challenges arise, we can accept them; and when we make mistakes, we can accept ourselves.

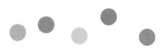

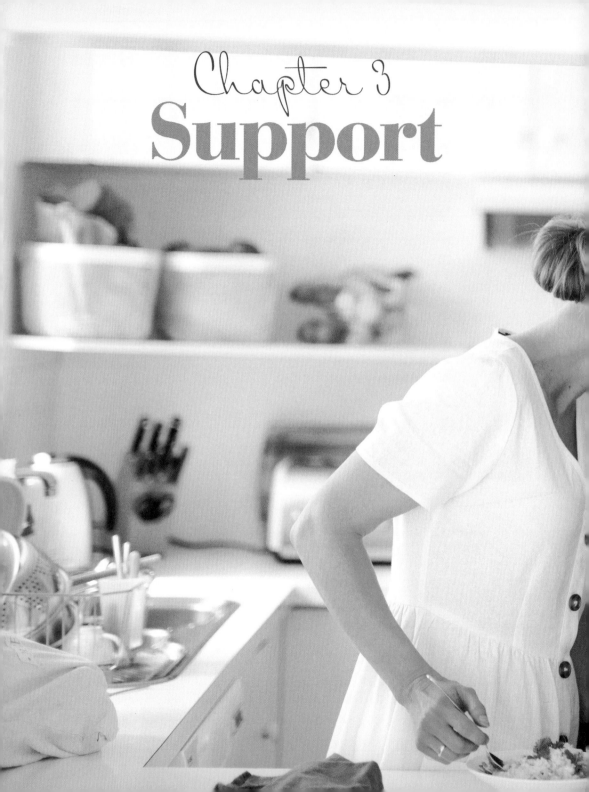

Chapter 3
Support

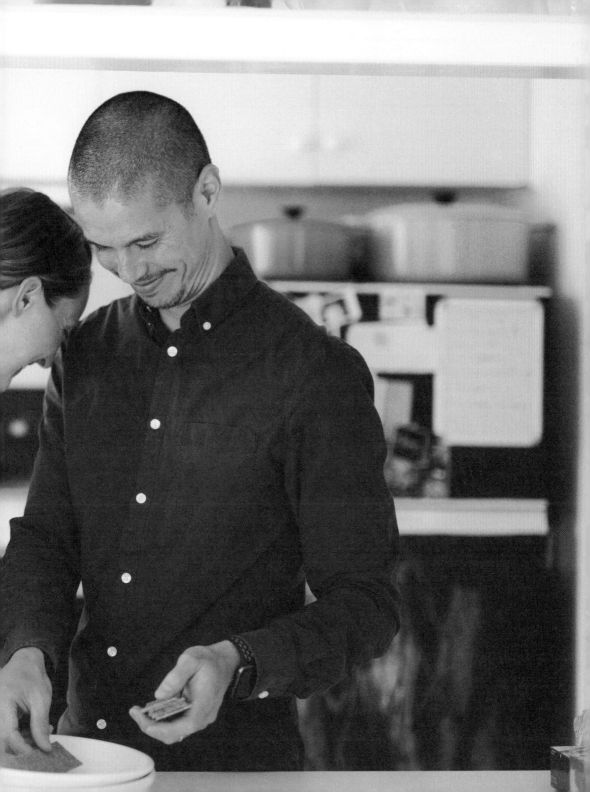

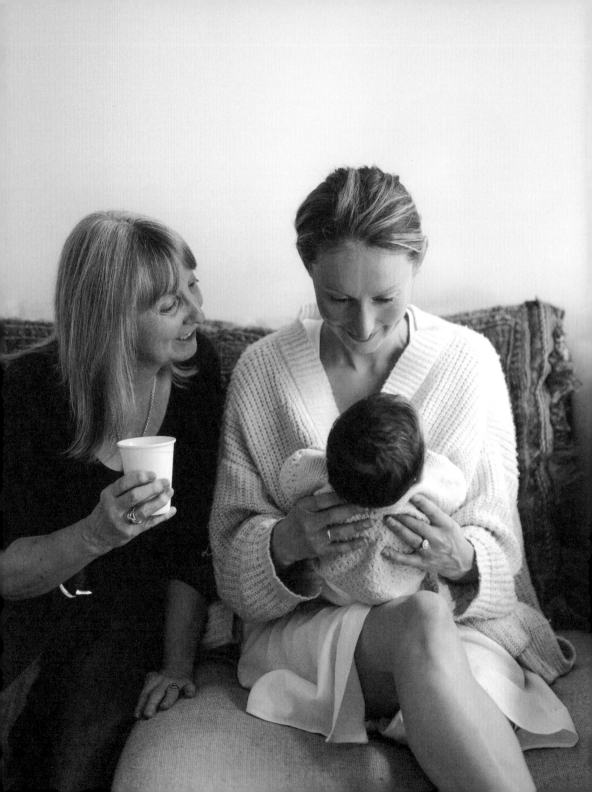

They're right. It really does take a village to provide a child with the care, companionship, wisdom and sense of belonging they need to thrive. In the early days, however, your baby will be content with just you. Your love, your touch, your nourishment are all they want. It will be you who'll need the care of your village. Intense and extraordinary changes occur within a woman when she nurtures new life, and the way she is supported, particularly in the initial days, weeks and months following childbirth, can greatly impact her mental and physical health. Cultures around the world continue to honour the tradition of confinement and care after birth, recognising it as a sacred and restorative time for mother and baby. Traditionally, this sees relatives taking over household chores and providing the new mother with sustenance, so that she can focus on her baby and herself. Western culture has forgone these practices, and yet mothers continue to require this sort of nurturing. In fact, with our inexperience, unrealistic expectations and relative isolation from family and friends – our village – it can be argued we need it more than ever.

Current research shows us the consequences of poor practical, social, financial and emotional support for new mothers. Not only is our physical recovery delayed or incomplete, we are left more vulnerable to postnatal mood disorders. At the very least, we become stretched thin as we struggle to do it all. In order to create the conditions for a gentle postnatal period, we need to be proactive in anticipating the sort of care we may require and mobilising the resources available to us. We need to patch together a village of sorts and not be afraid to reach out. This is our time to be nurtured.

Preparing for the birth

PREGNANCY AND CHILDBIRTH SUPPORT

All mothers, – particularly first-time mothers, for whom the experience of growing and birthing babies is entirely new – need to feel confident in the care they are receiving. They need to feel affirmed in the knowledge that pregnancy and childbirth are natural processes of which their body is entirely capable. They also need to feel that they are in good hands should they require medical intervention; because while pregnancy and childbirth are indeed natural processes, support is sometimes necessary to ensure mother and baby remain healthy. You may need to meet a number of midwives, obstetricians or other doctors before you find a person or team who makes you feel this way, and that's ok. Schedule appointments, seek answers to questions that are important to you and trust your intuition.

Depending on where you plan on giving birth, the sort of care available and your personal preferences, you may consider hiring a private midwife or doula for additional support. A private midwife will see you throughout your pregnancy and possibly attend your birth as an advocate and support person. They may also offer postnatal support. This is a great option for those wanting continuity of care. A doula is someone who is trained to provide you with physical and emotional support during pregnancy and childbirth (and possibly postnatally). This sort of non-medical support is tremendously important, and yet so lacking in our day and age. Good private midwives and doulas will be able to walk the fine line between de-medicalising the childbirth process, and encouraging you to be adaptable and accepting should medical intervention become necessary.

You may not need to hire someone to support and advocate for you and your baby in this way – an informed and sensitive partner, friend or relative can also play this role. Whoever you choose to be with you during labour and birth, keep in mind you need to feel relaxed and empowered, not fearful. Learning about childbirth and attending classes with your birth companion can help you feel this way and ensure you are both on the same page (more below). You may like to write a list of birth preferences to reinforce your wishes to your health care provider. Remember, though, that they are preferences and not a plan. You absolutely cannot plan your baby's birth, and it will serve you to accept this and be flexible.

BIRTHING CLASSES

Many first-time parents attend childbirth classes in the lead-up to their due date. I would encourage you to choose a class that aims to normalise the process and reduce any fear you may have about the birth of your child. HypnoBirthing and Calmbirth are two popular programs that work to empower parents-to-be in this manner and are valuable no matter where you plan on giving birth – at home, a birth centre or a hospital. These classes teach you and your birth companion how to help your body and baby work together during labour, thereby increasing your chance of a smooth delivery. This sort of information is incredibly beneficial, and would have traditionally been passed down by elders from your community. These classes also ensure you are aware of your options when birthing in a hospital setting, so that if you wish, you are equipped to avoid unnecessary interventions that may be suggested by health care providers out of convenience or extreme risk avoidance. You may feel happy with your standard hospital class and that's fine – just make sure you are left feeling as though your body was made to give birth, because that is precisely how you need to feel going into it.

Before the birth of our first child, Ben and I attended a HypnoBirthing course. I had always been interested in childbirth, but Ben had little knowledge on the subject. To him, birth was a woman lying on her back with her legs in the air, wearing a hospital gown, screaming and crippling her partner's hand – you know, the image portrayed in the movies. During our classes, Ben saw, for the first time ever, real footage of babies being born. He learned what the female body is capable of and, by having the process demystified, was able to relax his fears – which he otherwise would have brought into the labour environment, and which could have affected my ability to birth our child. He also learned ways to support me physically and emotionally throughout our birth experience, however it unfolded.

If you don't have the time or money to attend classes, reading books can also be beneficial (see page 310 for a list of suggested books). Just be sure to seek the answers to any questions you may have from qualified health professionals. Finally, you and your partner might also like to invest in classes that focus on the postnatal period, to learn how to care for your baby and each other.

A FINAL NOTE ON 'PREPARING' FOR BIRTH

Part of being well prepared for the birth of your baby involves being open to its unpredictable nature. You cannot possibly know how your baby's birth will unfold until it's happening, and it will serve you to surrender to that fact, and to trust your body, baby and midwife or other health care provider. As my wise friend Robin told me when I was fretting about the possibility of a c-section, at the end of the day, birth is about meeting your baby and becoming a mother, however that happens.

Preparing for postpartum life

CREATING A NEWBORN NEST

Most of the newborn days are spent feeding, sleeping and snuggling in your home. A comfortable, practical and clutter-free nest, with easy (one-handed) access to the things we need day to day, can help us feel content with the rhythm of our new life. But where do we begin? One of the most helpful things you can do when considering what baby items you may need is to walk through your house and role play the newborn days. Imagine feeding, changing and washing your baby; imagine helping them fall asleep; imagine caring for yourself. How can you help these acts flow with ease? When taking stock of your environment, you will find you don't need to invest in the most expensive, whizz-bang baby goods. Some items you will want to purchase, and that's fine, but you may also already have things on hand that you can repurpose, and all you will need to do is rearrange your space to suit your needs.

Feeding

Babies feed frequently and sometimes for a long time. You will need a comfortable place to sit while nourishing them. This may be your bed, a couch or a chair. Pillows can help to support your arms and back, and you can use a pillow designed specifically for breastfeeding or ones you already have around the house. If you're bottle-feeding, you will of course require bottles and items to ensure they are properly cleaned, as well as a pump and bags to freeze your milk, and/or formula. Make space for these items in your pantry and kitchen ahead of time, including space in your freezer for any expressed breastmilk.

Feeding time can be messy, so be sure to have cloths and bibs close by for you to grab. If you can, keep your feeding station well stocked with things for you, such as water, snacks, nipple cream and, when you've got feeding down pat and feel like tuning out, a book or TV remote.

Changing

You will also need somewhere to change your baby. Some people forgo the common baby change table purchase and opt for using a chest of drawers, their bed or the floor. Whatever you use, be sure it is safe and

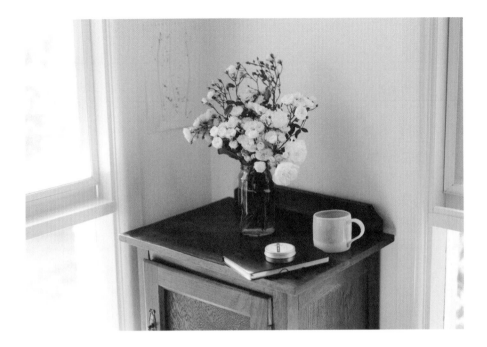

comfortable for your baby and yourself – you don't want to hurt your back by leaning over awkwardly multiple times a day – and never leave your baby unattended.

When changing your baby, you need to be able to grab wipes, cloths, water, nappies and creams or balm with ease (and possibly while holding a crying baby who has just done a poo explosion). Make sure these items are in a convenient place, such as a shelf on your change table or a nearby drawer. You will, of course, need to purchase these items. Though keep in mind that in early days, babies don't need wipes – warm water with a cloth will suffice (either a reusable cloth or disposable cotton pads). It's also a good idea to avoid creams that contain fragrances and parabens, as baby skin is super sensitive (see page 185 for more information).

Finally, you may like to decide whether you will use disposable or cloth nappies. Many find cloth is a good way to reduce the amount of waste they produce as a family. Do what works best for you and your baby, and know that you can always change your practice or use a combination of the two. It needn't be an all or nothing thing. Regardless of whether you use cloth nappies, you will need buckets for soaking clothes, and washing powder that is fragrance-free and gentle on baby skin.

Washing

Initially, babies don't need to be bathed often – a simple wipe with a cloth will do. The main thing to consider when deciding where and how to bathe your baby is, once again, safety and comfort. You need to be able to wash them with ease while keeping them safe. There are baby-specific baths you can purchase, but you may find you can do without one of these contraptions, provided you are organised (you don't want to be fumbling to find a towel or whatever you need when holding a wet baby, especially if you have bathed with them and are also wet).

Sleeping

Consider where your baby might sleep. Bassinets and moses baskets are popular options for the early days, or you may put your baby directly in a cot. You should also be prepared for the fact that your baby might prefer to sleep close to you at times, and borrow or buy a sling, wrap or baby carrier. That way, you can be respectful of their needs and get the benefit of skin-to-skin contact, while still being able to move about hands-free.

Swaddle blankets are a good way to help your baby feel safe and snug when it's time to sleep. It's worth buying a couple ahead of time and learning how to use them (ask a friend or your midwife, or watch some online tutorials). See Chapter 5: Sleep for more information.

Clothes and additional baby items

Your baby will need other things, such as clothes and a car seat. Bouncy chairs and prams are other purchases that can make your life easier. Where you can (and where appropriate), try to borrow items from friends. This will help you to avoid spending lots of money on clothes your baby will outgrow in a matter of days, or on items you may not end up using.

Your care

After you have considered how you will care for your newborn baby, think about how you will care for yourself. How you will ensure *you* are fed, clothed, bathed and rested? These are all important considerations when creating your newborn nest. Keep in mind you may have to do things one-handed on occasion, and avoid being on your feet for too long while you recover from childbirth.

YOUR HOME

In the season of new motherhood, it's easy to feel as though your whole life has been turned upside down. A clean and tidy home can help keep some order in your world. But completing the physical work of cleaning – and finding the time to do it – can be a challenge.

If you have the financial means, hiring someone to clean your house every so often is a decision you most certainly will not regret. Many postnatal doulas offer light housework as part of their service, along with food preparation and massage (yes, please!).

Alternatively, you may receive offers from supportive family members or friends who wish to pitch in. Here's the thing: *let them.* Forget that adorable onesie – a quick house-clean can be the best newborn present of all. A shoutout to my mother who cleaned our home while we were in the hospital with our newborn. If you are one of the first of your friends to have a baby, know that your friends may not recognise the value in doing dishes or folding laundry while they visit. I certainly didn't think to offer this help before becoming a mother. Ask them for a hand when they stop by. They will be pleased you did.

If you find yourself without cleaning assistance (and if scrubbing toilets isn't your definition of 'me time'), yet you still value a mess-free home, focus your attention on keeping just part of your house tidy. Identify where you spend most of your time – your living room and bedroom, perhaps? – and figure out a way to minimise mess. Keep rooms free of clutter by placing a basket in the corner, into which you can throw random items – a 'deal with it later' basket, if you will.

You might like to invest in an essential oil diffuser, along with some oils such as lavender, peppermint and citrus-based oils. This will do more than keep your home smelling fresh and inviting, as studies show essential oils can positively influence our mood and reduce anxiety. (Be sure to use essential oils safely, as discussed on page 135 – such as not on or close to young babies.) Natural light and fresh air also do wonders for your wellbeing, so remember to open the blinds and windows when you can.

PLAN YOUR SELF-CARE

Caring for yourself will help you continue caring your baby. See Chapter 4: Self-care for advice on the type of self-care you may benefit from, and how to fit it in when you have a newborn.

Nourishment

Good nourishment is essential in the perinatal period (that is, during and after pregnancy). And yet it's not always easy to obtain – particularly after birth, when our hands are full caring for our little one. New mothers need food that is nutrient dense, and easy to assemble and eat.

As part of your preparation for the newborn days, focus on nourishing your new-mother self. Ensure your pantry, fridge and freezer are well stocked with nutrient-rich foods that, with minimal effort, can be thrown together to make a meal or snack. I also recommend you call upon your village to bring you food after your baby is born. See chapters 6 and 7 for more advice on nourishing yourself.

OTHER PARENTS

Humans crave connection; it's one of our basic needs. Local councils arrange new parent groups in an attempt to foster social connectedness and minimise the feelings of isolation and loneliness that many report experiencing after birth. Whether you attend these sessions

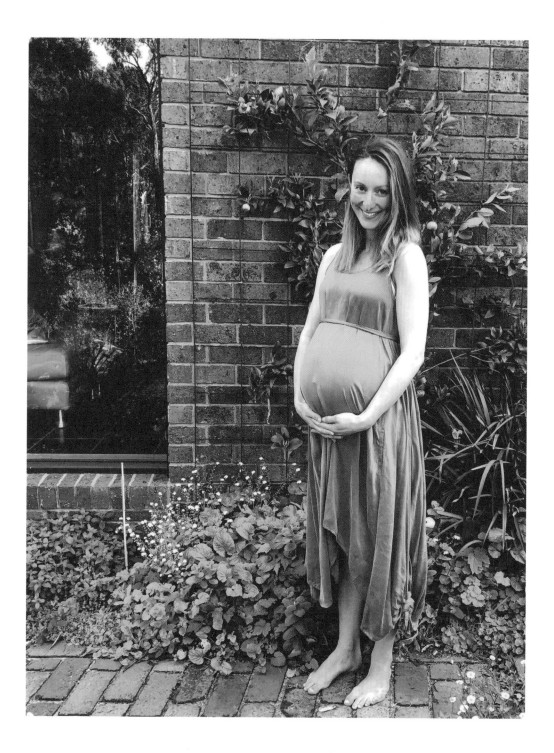

or find connection elsewhere, it's important to spend time with other parents, especially mothers. You may prefer to seek out women who are like-minded or broaden your horizons by connecting with those who approach life a little differently. Either way, the key is to seek out people who have babies born at a similar time. While mothers of older children can be wise and wonderfully supportive, our memory of the realities of this season can fade with time and, as a result, we run the risk of over-romanticising the newborn days.

New parents commonly hear that this is 'the best time', when what they may actually need is validation that this is a hard time. People with babies of similar ages will understand this because they are also in the thick of it. If you don't have friends with babies, try a council-run parents' group or local online group. It may take time to find people you click with, so be aware of that. You may also find comfort and connection with mothers on the other side of the world through social media. Just be sure to follow people who share the realities of motherhood and not just the picture-perfect moments.

PROFESSIONAL SUPPORT

Physiotherapist

A woman's health physiotherapist can help you strengthen your pelvic floor during and after pregnancy, and assist with the management of complications such incontinence and prolapse. Even if you had a smooth pregnancy and delivery, it's a good idea to get checked out and learn how to best support your recovery. This is especially important if you plan to engage in vigorous physical activity (which, by the way, isn't a good idea for most women in the initial months following birth). It takes time for your body to recover from growing and birthing a baby. Patience and proper care will help you get there.

Lactation consultant and breastfeeding support

Learning to feed your baby can be a challenging, painful and emotionally exhausting process. If you wish to breastfeed, the way the early days and weeks unfold, and the support you receive, can mean the difference between continuing and stopping before you hoped.

Hopefully you will receive good support from your midwives or a lactation consultant after birth. If you don't, or even if you do, you may wish to consider booking an appointment with a lactation consultant in the initial days or week. A voucher for a home visit would make a great baby shower present. At the very least, put the number of a consultant and the Australian Breastfeeding Association on your fridge so you can contact them if you have any questions or concerns.

You should never be made to feel that breastfeeding is something to hide, so try to surround yourself with those who are supportive of your desire to breastfeed your baby – however long you choose to do so. It's a glorious act, with immeasurable health and bonding benefits.

Paediatrician

Babies get coughs, rashes and things you never knew existed, like cradle cap. Instead of searching for answers online, it's better for your baby's health and your peace of mind to seek the advice of a qualified health professional. Check out local doctors before your baby arrives and find one whose health care philosophies match your own. That way, when your baby gets sick, you won't be scrambling to find a doctor at the last minute.

Counsellor

Seeking a counsellor to support you and your partner throughout the perinatal period is a sensible idea. This is especially important if you had a traumatic birth experience, are struggling to sleep, if you simply don't feel like yourself and if you have a history of mental health issues (though it must be said, not everyone who has a history of mental health issues will experience a recurrence or exacerbation of symptoms).

Try to make appointments ahead of time for the weeks following birth (ideally with a counsellor who works with women in the perinatal period). Even if you're feeling fairly emotionally stable, being able to talk about your experiences can make a big difference to your adjustment and overall wellbeing.

FINANCIAL SUPPORT

Before your baby arrives, find out the types of governmental financial support that may be available to you as a new parent. While the act of raising future generations is undoubtedly undervalued, many countries do offer a small amount of money to assist families in the postnatal period. After the birth you may have foggy baby-brain, so you may wish to ask your partner, family or friends to help with submitting the necessary paperwork and registering your baby's birth to get the payments flowing.

If you are presently employed, learn about the parental leave options your current workplace may offer. You and your partner might be entitled to a certain amount of pay on top of any government support. Super-savvy parents might consider starting a postnatal fund before they even conceive, in order to reduce financial pressure and make it possible for one or more parent to take extended time off work, if that is what they desire.

RETURNING TO WORK

In addition to finding out your financial entitlements from your current workplace, you might like to find out how flexible it is with regard to your return date, payment structure, working hours and working location.

For example, you may be permitted to extend the length of your leave at reduced pay, which can allow you to remain home for longer with your baby and avoid childcare costs. In addition, you might be able to arrive at work earlier (or later) than usual and/or leave earlier (or later) than usual. You may also be permitted to work from home some of the time. It pays, pun most certainly intended, to make the most of the opportunities available to you.

If your options are limited, there is value in initiating a dialogue about the benefits of flexible working arrangements for parents. Many companies recognise this and, in order to retain valued staff and reduce turnover, are beginning to offer their employees greater flexibility. Find out what your employer is open to, while informing them of your earnest desire to do a good job both at work and home.

OR NOT RETURNING TO WORK

It's not uncommon for a parent to change their mind about returning to work after the baby arrives (and, it must be said, it's also not uncommon to be excited about returning to work). If, for whatever reason, you believe it's not in your family's best interests for you and/or your partner to work outside the home in your previous role(s), you will hopefully have some options that will allow you to follow your intuition.

It's worth noting, though, that even if you do feel the pull to stay home, and are able to do so, it may not be an easy decision. Depending on your field of work, hitting pause on your career could very well require you to make significant sacrifices regarding your career progression. Only you will know if this is a sacrifice you're willing to make. You may like to seek out other parents who have made this decision; their circumstances will be different, but they will surely have some valuable insights.

Take a good look at your budget to see if you can make adjustments to your spending that will allow your family to survive on a reduced income. You might cut down your food expenditure or holidays, or you might consider moving to a more affordable area (though you will need to consider the implications of leaving any community support you might have). If you rely on a double income, consider finding more flexible or part-time work, or work you can do from home. Whatever your decision, the reality is that it may not be ideal; sacrifices will surely need to be made. But if it allows you to do what want – that is, to be home with your baby more than you would have been – then you will probably feel it's worth it.

Lastly, know that while you may not earn a paycheque from being a stay-at-home parent, raising a healthy, resilient, kind, empathetic and emotionally aware individual is invaluable work.

CHILDCARE

If you are unable to care for your child full-time – say, if you want or need to return to work, or if you are unwell – you and your partner will need to think about who you might enlist to take on this role.

Your partner or family

First, consider whether your partner can stop work or reduce their workload. Indeed, the care shouldn't fall entirely to the mother (though it's easy to see how this happens if you are exclusively breastfeeding). Have your partner assess their work flexibility, and if they cannot take on this role, you might be able to ask a willing family member for assistance. There are pros and cons to the latter option, so be sure to weigh them up and see whether it is a good fit for you, both emotionally and financially.

If you do have family available to pitch in, it can be immensely beneficial to utilise them, even for a brief time. A friend of mine had a kind aunty who was willing to be on standby for emergencies, such as when her baby was sick and couldn't attend childcare during the time when my friend was transitioning back to work.

If family do become involved, no doubt concessions will need to be made by both parties in order to preserve your relationship – in other words, you will need to pick your battles.

Daycare centres, in-home care and nannies

You might also consider more formal childcare options, such as daycare. When choosing a centre for your child, think about whether you prefer it to be close to your home or your workplace. Daycare spots book up in advance, so this is something you may want to think about early on; frequently, expectant parents begin the search well before the baby is born, and put their name on a waiting list (or lists) to ensure they secure a spot. Tour a number of facilities to learn about their training and policies, and get a feel for the environment and staff. Always use your intuition when making a decision; if you have a gut feeling about a place, don't dismiss your instincts.

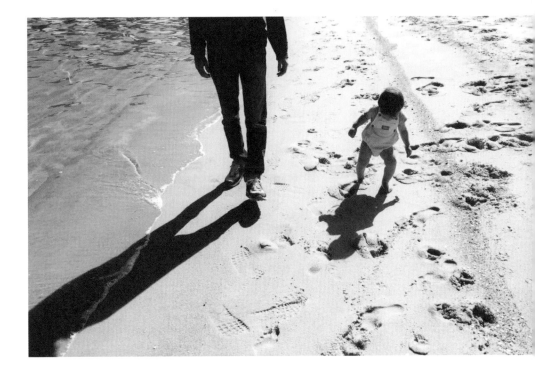

Other options include in-home daycare or hiring a nanny, whether to care for your child alone or to share with another family. The nanny option can be appealing, as babies benefit from one-on-one attention and the opportunity to develop a close bond with their carer (and while this bond can also be found in a daycare setting, it's arguably easier to achieve with a nanny). There are, however, drawbacks to this arrangement, including an often increased financial cost and the reliance on a single individual (who may occasionally have to call in sick).

When children get older, many parents like the daycare option as it allows children to socialise (though it must be said, there are other ways children can socialise). Returning to work and/or changing caregivers will always be a big transition for both parent and child, so give it time and be compassionate.

Perinatal mood disorders

The myriad changes and challenges that occur during pregnancy and in the postnatal period (collectively known as the perinatal period) place our mental health in a vulnerable position. Research tells us that the number of women who experience depression and/or anxiety during pregnancy is one in ten, rising to one in seven after birth. One in ten partners will also experience mood disorder symptoms in the postnatal period. The reason these complications develop are individual and generally categorised as being of biological nature (i.e., the huge hormonal shifts that occur during this period), psychological nature (i.e., a previous history of mental illness) and social nature (i.e., poor support or a recent triggering event). Throw in the common postnatal realities of sleep deprivation, a monumental change in identity and perhaps suboptimal nourishment, and you can appreciate why mood disorders are a reality for so many parents.

In fact, the number of people who experience these issues is probably higher than the current reported levels, as depression and anxiety so often go undetected and untreated. It is crucial, then, that we understand the prevalence of perinatal mood disorders and know the symptoms, so that women, partners and other support people are in a better place to recognise if they, or someone they know, develop one.

In the days following childbirth, when our baby and placenta have left our body, our hormone levels drop dramatically. Most new mothers will experience what is called the 'baby blues', feeling sensitive, teary, moody and/or flat. In many cases, these symptoms subside within a week or so. In the case of postnatal depression, they will persist and may get worse.

Every woman's experience with postnatal depression is different: common symptoms include difficulty concentrating, sleeping or bonding with their baby; feeling perpetually lonely, hopeless and fatigued; and a change in appetite. Many communities screen new mothers for postnatal depression, but this relies on the woman being able to recognise what is going on and share her feelings. When you're in the thick of it, this can be hard to do. In addition, not everyone's experience will fit into the cultural perception of a mood disorder – that is, a person feeling sad and crying all the time.

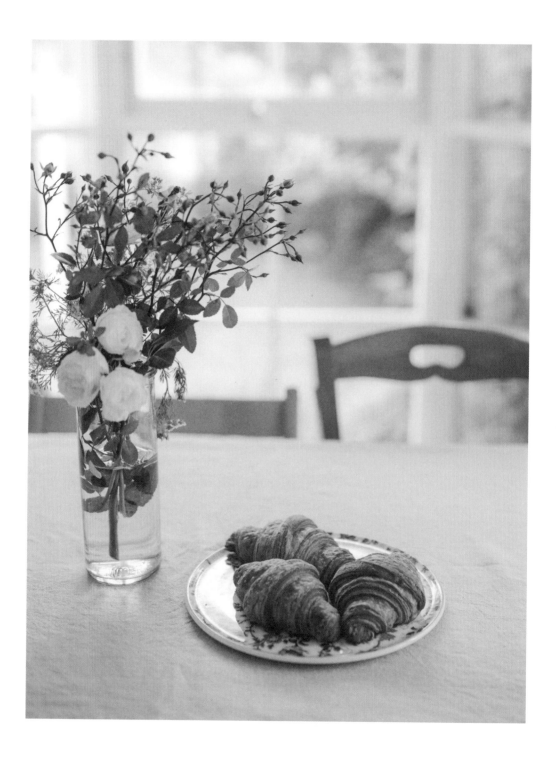

In the case of perinatal anxiety, anxious thoughts and feelings occupy the woman's mind and body, which can leave her feeling jittery (i.e., the opposite of flat). While it's normal to be on high alert, as our protective, mother-bear instincts kick in, if these anxious thoughts become persistent and intrusive – and inhibit the mother's ability to sleep, eat, care for her baby, feel content and just generally function as she normally would – they need addressing.

Beyond having anxious thoughts, a woman may experience panic attacks and/or develop obsessive and compulsive tendencies, feeling the need to perform certain rituals in order to achieve a certain outcome (often to stop bad things from happening). Mothers, and their partners, can also develop post-traumatic stress disorder, commonly triggered by a traumatic birth experience.

Finally, though rare, a new mother may develop postnatal psychosis, which will see her disconnect from reality, possibly with hallucinations and episodes of mania. This places her at risk of harming herself and her baby, and requires urgent action, including hospitalisation.

The postnatal period can be incredibly challenging. Sometimes these challenges cause women to experience symptoms of a mood disorder, yet with proper social support, these can be managed. Sleep deprivation is one example: if the mother is allowed to get more sleep, her mental health often improves.

Depending on the severity of a mother's symptoms, more intensive treatment, including medication, is required. While some women are hesitant to take medication, there are options available that are deemed safe to consume while pregnant and breastfeeding. Furthermore, research suggests that untreated maternal depression and anxiety can be of greater risk to babies than the actual medication. Regardless of whether medication is required, counselling should be a part of a care plan, as well as being checked for nutritional deficiencies, such as vitamin D and iron, and supplementing accordingly. Omega-3 DHA and probiotic supplements may very well be beneficial, too.

It is also crucial that women in the perinatal period receive adequate nourishment from food, and not just supplements. Yet because mood disorders tend to alter our appetite, many women struggle to eat enough and will need support to assist them (more in chapters 6 and 7). There are other things to monitor, such as thyroid function and activity level. Abnormal thyroid levels are not uncommon after pregnancy, and it is well known that being active is incredibly beneficial for mental health. Other complementary therapies, such as acupuncture, can also be helpful.

I appreciate this sounds like an exhaustive list, but there are many reasons why a mood disorder will thrive, and different things may help different women. If you are presently dealing with a perinatal mood disorder, know that it's normal to believe you won't ever feel like yourself again. Many women feel this way. But with treatment, support and time they get there, and so will you.

If a mood disorder becomes a part of your motherhood experience, be gentle on yourself, and remember you are not alone. In fact, considering the statistics, it's likely you know someone who has been through, or is going through, a similar struggle. Be sure to check in, then – with yourself and your parent friends. **Note:** See page 310–11 for where to find mental health support.

You and your partner

In writing this next section, I have made a few assumptions. I have assumed you have a partner who lives in the same house as you, and who is physically and emotionally present throughout your pregnancy and postnatal experience. I acknowledge this is not always the case – some women do not have this kind of support, or they might receive it from a friend or relative instead of their partner. If this is your experience, my hope is the next section will still provide you with insight as to the kind of support you may desire and benefit from during this time.

If you do have a present partner, know that this section is as much for them as it is for you – so, bookmark the page for them when you're done. Many partners report feeling useless during pregnancy, childbirth and the early days, but the truth is, they are far from useless. In fact, their involvement and support can make the world of difference to your experience, while also helping them to bond with their baby and embrace their new role as a parent with confidence.

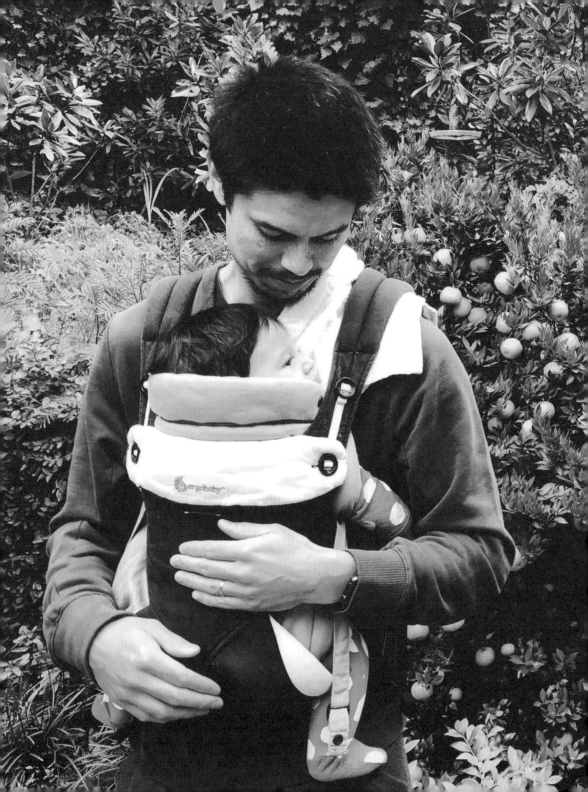

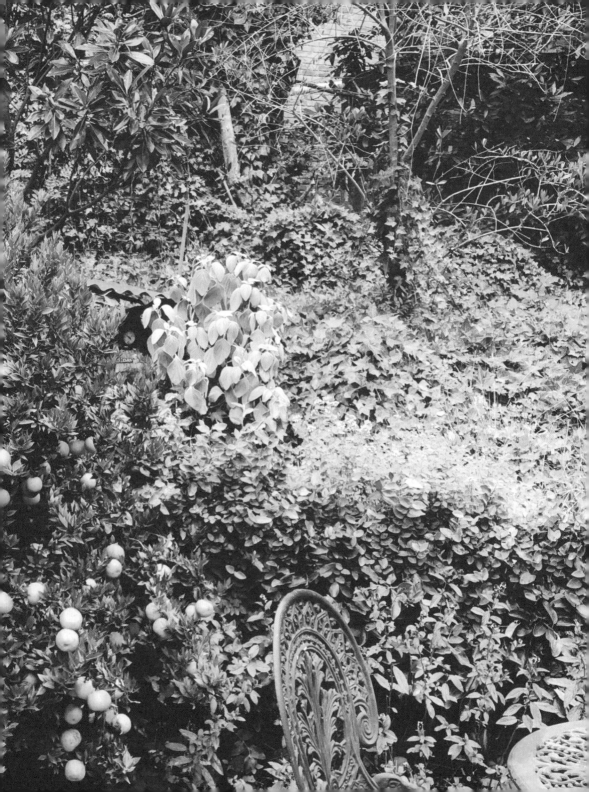

Pregnancy support

Your partner may be able to support you, and feel connected to your growing baby, during pregnancy by:

- attending appointments

- feeling the baby kick and talking to the baby

- massaging your body

- assembling the bassinet, change table, and so on

- discussing baby names

- reading books about birth and newborn life (see pages 310–12)

- attending birth classes

- helping to declutter and clean your home

- investigating the type of leave they can take from work and looking into flexible work options

- helping to stock the freezer with meals for the newborn days.

Share how you're feeling with your partner – from how it feels to physically grow your baby, to any hopes or concerns you may have for the birth and postnatal period.

Childbirth support

While you are in labour, your partner may be able to support you by:

- ensuring your bags are packed and in the car, if giving birth away from home, and by being prepared in case a trip to a hospital or birthing centre is required unexpectedly

- ensuring the car has enough petrol to get where you're going

- knowing where you're going and keeping an eye on roadworks or closures along your route

- helping you to feel safe, relaxed and loved

- checking in and asking you what you want or need

- preparing any food and beverages you desire

- playing any music you may want

- running the bath or shower for you, and helping you get in and out safely

- massaging your body and using acupressure points

- giving you positive affirmations

- communicating with midwives and other health care providers, and advocating for your birth preferences

- continuing to be a pillar of strength and support, no matter how the birth unfolds or progresses (i.e., not freaking out when unexpected things occur, and not taking it personally if the mother communicates in a short and snappy way)

- checking in with how they are feeling and getting support from midwives if required. Birth is a big deal and it's understandable your partner may have a lot of emotions or thoughts running through their mind, yet they need to not let their feelings impact you or the birthing process

- when appropriate, and if they wish, helping to deliver their baby (i.e., being the one to 'catch' their baby and passing the baby to you after birth), announcing the gender and cutting the umbilical cord.

Postnatal support

The type of support you require after birth will vary depending on your experience, though your partner might be able to help by:

- making and bringing you nourishment

- holding their baby so you can sleep, rest, shower, eat and do other forms of self-care

- cleaning the house

- doing the laundry

- participating in settling their baby

- participating in bottle-feeding, if that's what you're doing

- asking how you are feeling, and being patient and present while you talk (without necessarily trying to fix anything)

- looking out for signs of mood disorders, without freaking out any time you get teary; remember, it's normal to have a bit of baby blues

- making sure you don't have too many visitors and that they don't stay too long – 20 minutes is a good limit, though feel free to make it even shorter

- telling you that you are doing a wonderful job, that your baby is so lucky to have you as a mother, and that you are loved.

You might be able to support your partner in the postnatal period by:

- sharing what you're going through – any struggles, any feelings of gratitude

- giving them bonding time with their baby. Encourage them to put skin to skin, as it can increase your partner's oxytocin levels and lower their cortisol levels, which can help them develop a stronger attachment and feel less stressed

- allow them to care for their baby without jumping to tell them the 'right' way to do things

- telling your partner they are doing a wonderful job, that their baby is so lucky to have them as a parent, that they are making such a difference to how you feel and that they are loved.

ADJUSTING TO PARENTHOOD AS A COUPLE

The first year of parenthood is hard on relationships. Research shows that the majority of married couples report a decrease in marital satisfaction and overall happiness in the year after their baby is born. Knowing this, it's wise for expectant couples to consider counselling throughout the perinatal period. At the very least, you will want to sit down together before your baby arrives and get on the same page regarding the kind of support you each anticipate needing, as well as what you expect of each other in terms of baby care and household duties.

If you do see a counsellor, a follow-up session once your baby arrives will allow you to work through any issues that may have cropped up, including unexpected challenges (of which there can be many). Perhaps you feel as though you can do without counselling, and that's fine – the important thing is to connect and communicate.

The more open you are with each other, the easier it will be for you to support each other as your family grows. In reality, this is easier said than done. Because as you are going through the significant transition of becoming a parent, neither of you will be getting adequate sleep – which is to say there will probably be a lot of feelings floating around, and you may, at times, be sensitive and snappy.

Clear and respectful communication of your feelings and needs, and not expecting your partner to read your mind, can help ensure you get the practical and emotional support you require. It can also help you to feel compassion, rather than resentment, for each other, and minimise tension. This is important at all times, though especially when you become parents, as your interactions will influence your child's sense of security and provide vital modelling for their future relationships.

When my husband transitioned back to work, I found myself feeling angry when he would return home distracted or grumpy. Eventually we realised that we needed to be more open with each other. Once he began sharing what was on his mind, I was able to understand what he was going through and more easily feel compassion for him (and vice versa). Though it sounds simple, this is something we still have to remind ourselves to do when life gets busy.

Another thing you can do to nurture your relationship is try to incorporate little acts of connection in your everyday lives – whether it's picking your partner a flower from the garden, dancing together in the kitchen to your favourite song, filling up a hot water bottle and putting it in their bed at night, or looking them in the eye and verbally expressing your gratitude when they do something kind. These gestures say a lot and can help you and your partner to feel as though you are on the same team.

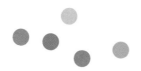

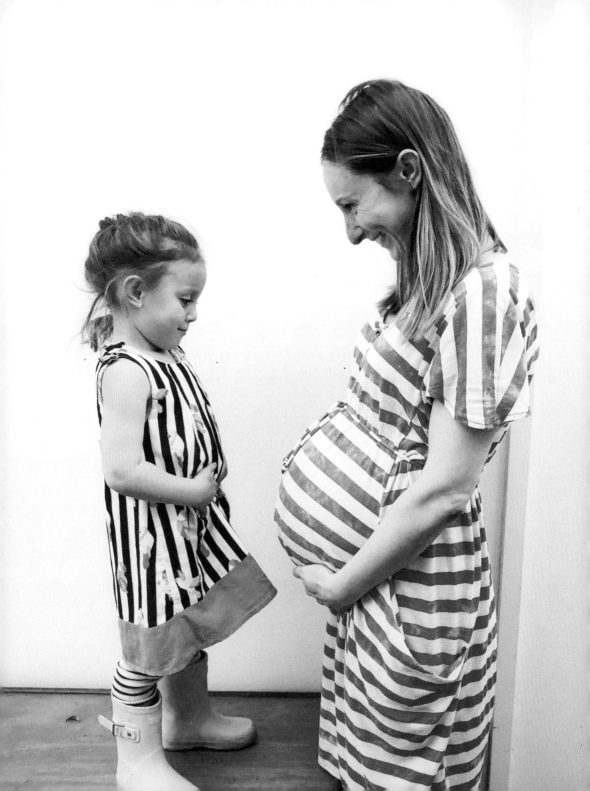

Chapter 4
Self-care

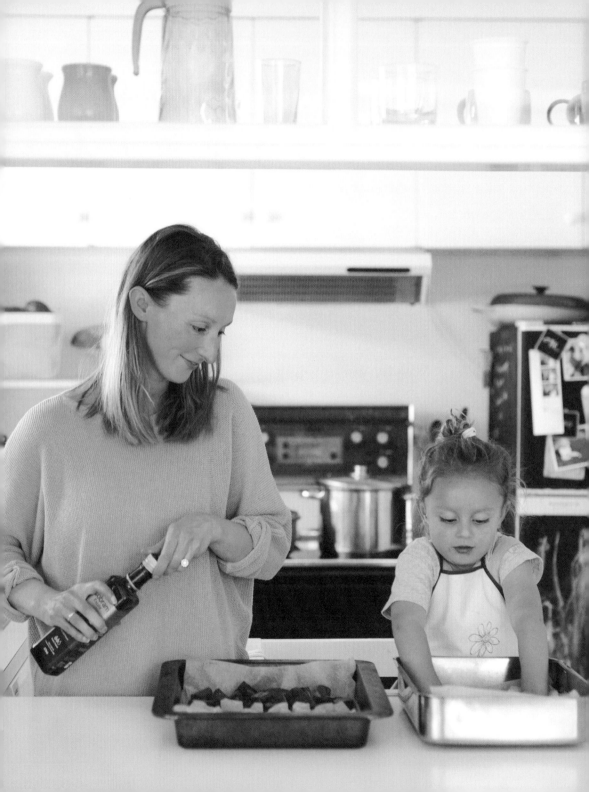

When I was at around 35 weeks pregnant with Walt and preparing, once again, to enter into the newborn bubble, people began asking me what I was going to do differently this time around. My response was simple: 'I'm focusing less on my baby and more on myself.' Sure, I'd dusted off the bassinet and washed baby clothes, but mostly I spent time gathering personal items for my nest, cooking and freezing meals, and rearranging my home and schedule so that I could be as comfortable and fortified as possible after the birth. Because I now knew that babies don't need stuff, they need you. And when you feel nurtured, it is easier to embrace their dependence rather than resist or resent it.

Fitting in self-care when you're busy caring for your baby may feel like a luxury, but the truth is, it's a necessity and should be treated as such. Growing and nurturing new life requires you to give greatly of yourself, and in order to continue giving, you need to replenish your body and mind by intentionally weaving acts of care into the demanding newborn days (and beyond).

When you become a mother, self-care will clearly look a little different from how it did before. You won't have the same time allowance as you previously did, and whatever act you do may not have the same effect as it used to. By this I mean, there's a good chance you won't feel completely rejuvenated by your self-care practices. That's ok, though. Accepting the season you're in can help reduce the expectation that you should be feeling marvellous all the time, or that self-care will fix everything, because that isn't a realistic goal. The result may just be that you feel a bit better than you did beforehand or that you've prevented yourself from becoming entirely depleted – both of which are good and worthy goals.

Your practice needn't involve large chunks of time or money, either. During this time, completing even basic acts, such as showering and eating, can be a challenge (surprisingly so). Think small, then, and focus on the things you can do each day to feel nurtured. When taking a shower no longer requires divine timing, you may like to expand your repertoire; but in the beginning, it's the little acts of care, such as those described in this chapter, that are the most powerful and restorative.

Before becoming a mother, caring for myself required little forethought. I was easily and often able to do my basic acts of self-care, in addition to those that were more time-intensive and extravagant. In fact, at the time, I don't think I would ever have called showering, eating and moving 'self-care'. It was only when my baby arrived, and my ability to do these things changed, that I realised how essential they were to my wellbeing. When I neglected to care for myself in these ways, my head felt foggier, my energy levels and mood were lower, and my struggles felt greater. I didn't feel anywhere near as content with my world. And so, I made it a priority to care for myself in the most basic and beneficial of ways.

I used the approximate 3 minutes per day that Joan was happy outside of my arms to shower and stretch; I made sure to plan ahead so I would have feel-good food available to me throughout the day; and during one of her naps, I'd pop her in a baby carrier and walk around the neighbourhood. As Joan grew, it became easier to complete these acts and incorporate new ones, too, such as writing and spending time with friends – both of which helped me to feel like a whole person.

When pondering how to care for yourself, consider where you're at – what is necessary and achievable in your present stage? On the following pages is a list of self-care practices many women find essential and revitalising during pregnancy and the newborn days. Use it as a prompt to find what works for you. Once you have tuned in and know the sort of care you need, the next step is to incorporate it into your life with reverence. When you are devoted to your wellbeing, you are far more likely to find pockets of time throughout the day where you can care for yourself.

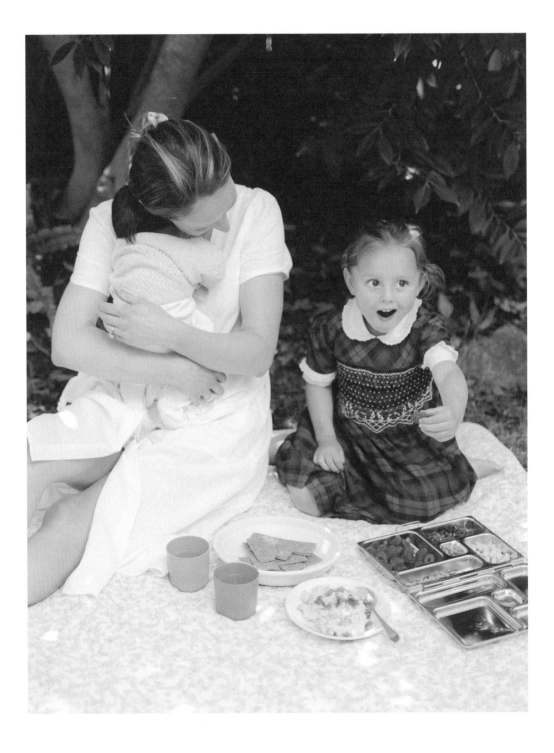

Self-care suggestions

FEED YOURSELF

In order for your body and mind to function well, and in order to grow and nourish your baby, you need to feed yourself. While this may sound easy enough, it's often not. You may experience pregnancy-related symptoms that impede your ability to eat, or you may simply be too busy caring for your newborn. Chances are that during this time the simple act of nourishing yourself may require more effort that you're used to. Thus, I have included feeding yourself as a form of self-care. Add it to your list, along with drinking plenty of water, and see chapters 6 and 7 for more advice.

PREPARE FOOD

In busy seasons of life, preparing food ahead of time can mean the difference between eating a nutrient-rich meal, and either not eating anything or eating something lacklustre. Many parents find food preparation a saviour in the postnatal period. You may also benefit from the practice during pregnancy, say, if you find yourself working long hours or feeling too tired to cook in the evenings. See pages 220–3 for more information on food preparation.

SHOWER OR BATHE

Bathing or showering in warm water can help relieve tension, ease anxiety and even increase your oxytocin levels. This can be immensely helpful to ease back pain associated with pregnancy, or to relax your body during labour. In the newborn days (and beyond), a rush of water over your body can be outstandingly invigorating, helping to clear the fog. A shower tends to be more achievable than a bath, but many people find a warm bath sits right at the top of their self-care list. If that's the case for you, figure out a way to fit baths in, such as when your baby is asleep or your partner is home. You can even bathe with your baby – the experience will be a little different, but you and your baby will get the benefit of warm water and skin-to-skin contact.

STRETCH

Another simple and effective way to energise your body is to stretch. Pregnancy and caring for a newborn can create all sort of aches and pains, and a good stretch can help relieve tension. It can also improve your mood and strengthen your mind–body connection.

During pregnancy, your body produces a hormone that causes your ligaments to relax. As a result you may find you are bendier than usual, so stick to gentle stretches to avoid injury. Start with stretching your arms and legs as wide as possible before you get out of bed in the morning. As the day moves along, find little moments here and there to stretch and move your body. This will be especially valuable if you get stuck in one position for an extended period, as can happen easily when breastfeeding or holding a sleeping baby. A few yoga poses can do the trick. Slow down and gently lean into whatever feels good in your body in that moment.

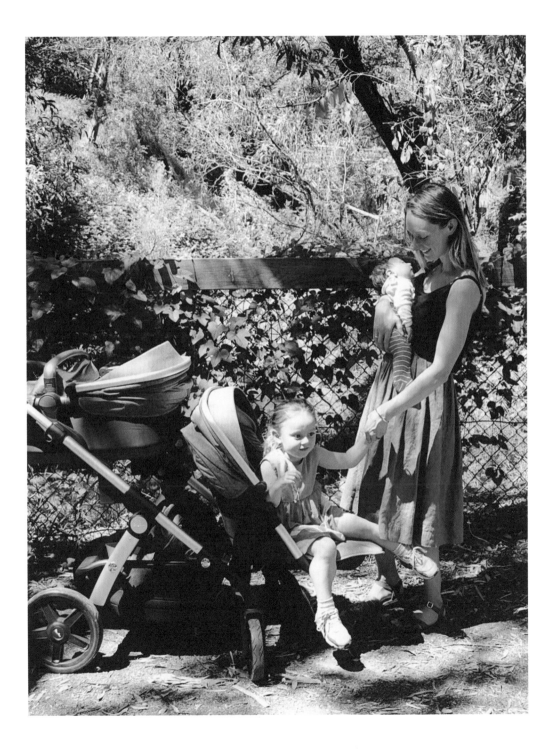

MOVE

When we move our body, we receive both instantaneous and long-lasting benefits. Whether it's walking, swimming or stretching, movement improves our energy levels and sleep quality, as well as our overall mental and physical health. If we remain active when pregnant, our risk of experiencing certain complications is reduced. Research suggests we can even improve our baby's health outcomes. Another benefit of being active during pregnancy is that it might encourage an easier and faster labour and recovery.

Whenever you feel like you can't be bothered with a walk or stretch session when you're tired, try to remember these benefits and do what you can. Even a few minutes will make a difference. If you're unsure what sort of movement feels good to you, seek the advice of an exercise professional who works with women in the perinatal period. Check you're not doing anything too strenuous during pregnancy by seeing whether you can talk through your movements – generally speaking, it's ok to exert yourself, but you should still be able to talk. Pilates is a wonderful option that can strengthen and support your muscles as your body goes through a truly amazing transformation.

Keep in mind, though, that you don't need to put on active gear or do a formal class to get your body moving. Walking is free and wonderfully energising. If you can move outdoors, you will get the benefit of fresh air and, on sunny days, a hit of vitamin D. Sometimes, especially soon after birth, you may find wriggling your bare toes on the ground is all the movement you need.

REST

Just as movement is beneficial for our wellbeing, so too is rest. While you are growing and caring for babies, rest is often the best thing you can do for yourself – particularly in the days after childbirth, and when your baby is going through periods of night waking. Tune in and notice when your body needs rest and, when you can, allow it to – whether you actually take a nap or simply lie down.

MOISTURISE AND MASSAGE

As your body changes its size and shape, and as your hormones fluctuate, you may find your skin benefits from a little extra care. Moisturising and massaging won't 'fix' all of the changes you might see in your skin (indeed, it appears that hereditary factors determine whether or not we develop stretch marks), but these practices can help you to feel more connected to, and comfortable in, your body. They can also alleviate dry spots, relieve tension, improve circulation and even have a positive impact on your mental health.

When choosing a moisturiser, look for an oil or cream that is free of fragrances and parabens (more on page 185), and place it on your bathroom bench as a reminder to feed your skin. While you're at it, treat yourself to a nice hand cream (dry hands are common in the postnatal period). Many women like to treat themselves to pregnancy and postnatal massages, to really take care of those aches and pains and encourage relaxation. If this isn't on the cards for you, a quick massage from your partner can be beneficial. It's also a nice way to connect with each other when you may not feel like being intimate in other ways.

CONSIDER YOUR WARDROBE

This may seem like an odd form of self-care, but hear me out. Culturally, we don't embrace body changes – particularly when it involves enlarging or softening. Yet over the course of our life as a woman, our body will experience significant growth and change, most notably during and after pregnancy. One thing we can do to help us accept our changing body and treat it with kindness is ensure we have access to feel-good clothes. By this I mean items we can easily throw on and feel confident and comfortable in.

Many women tend to do a good job of embracing the bump during pregnancy with maternity clothing, only to find themselves at a loss postnatally. It's wise to plan ahead and prepare a few items for the season after pregnancy, as this is when women often feel most dissatisfied with their body. Big and breathable underwear, stretchy pants, soft cotton tops, button-down shirts and loose dresses are comfortable and practical for recovery and breastfeeding. It can be helpful to create a mini-wardrobe of these sorts of clothes, as it will allow you to select items without fuss, and without seeing all the things you can no longer fit into.

I recognise that clothing choice is a privileged matter, but it undeniably has the power to influence our contentment and help us stay in the realm of acceptance and positivity – and not solely for women who are prone to body dissatisfaction. Think of how pleasurable it feels to slip into a soft robe or cosy jumper. When you're up feeding at night or getting dressed for your day after 3 broken hours of sleep, you want your clothes to summon that feeling, instead of, 'Oomph, nothing fits.'

CONNECT

Research has shown that feeling connected to others and having positive social relationships is fundamental to our wellbeing. Social connectedness can reduce our risk of anxiety and depression, enhance our empathy and strengthen our immune system.

These days, we are able to connect readily to people via mobile phones and social media, which is certainly helpful in combating isolation. However, we don't necessarily partake in as many of the day-to-day, face-to-face interactions which are vital to our health and happiness.

People lead busy lives, drop-in visits are a rarity and many of us don't know our neighbours the way we used to. Thus, we may need to schedule regular catch-ups with friends and family in order to get that connection buzz. When going through periods of significant transition, it's helpful to connect with those who can sympathise and appreciate what you are experiencing and validate your feelings. Therefore, you may find yourself wanting to spend more time with your pregnant and new-parent friends. Or you may gravitate towards people who aren't in your life stage, so you can take a break from baby talk.

When Joan was around 4 months old, I found myself scheduling our daily walk to coincide with the local school drop-off or pick-up, as this allowed me to chat with the crossing guard. This 70-year-old man was certainly not a new mother, and our conversation rarely extended beyond a friendly hello or talk of the weather, but it was precisely what I needed.

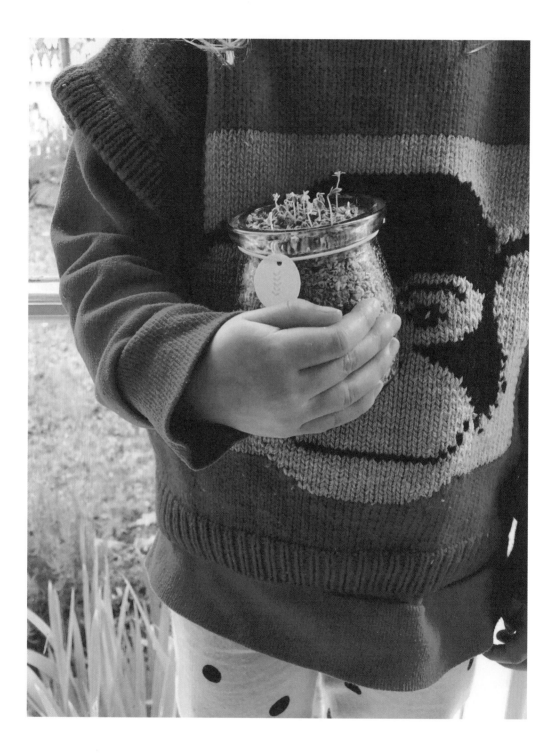

On a slightly different note, I also found podcasts helped satisfy my desire for connection – even though it was a one-sided interaction. Most days I popped one on and made sure to listen to shows that covered a range of topics, not just motherhood.

CLEAN HOUSE

Cleaning or tidying your home may seem like a boring form of self-care, but sometimes it is just the thing you need to do to feel content. A good scrub can be a form of movement, too, and you can always listen to music or a podcast while you do it.

WRITE

In the early months after Joan's birth, I would spend her nap time writing. Becoming a mother brought momentous change to my world and, as a long-time journaller, writing was my way of processing this. I wrote about her birth, our life, my thoughts and my feelings, and in doing so was able to release the jumble of thoughts from my head and acknowledge my feelings – both the positive and negative ones. Not all of our feelings about this time will be positive, and it is important to find a healthy way to express them. For me, that looks like writing.

GET A HEALTH CHECK UP

Visiting a counsellor, physiotherapist or other health care professional may not be the most enjoyable form of self-care, but at times it may be the most important. After Walt's birth, my appointments with a woman's health physiotherapist were crucial in helping me to feel strong and good in my body.

Actually doing it

After identifying the practices that fill up your cup, the next step is to do them. Make sure what you are proposing is achievable in your present circumstances, and then figure out how you might be able to work the practice into your day. It's likely you won't need guidance on how to do this in the time before your baby arrives, which is why this next section will focus on the postnatal period. Take a look at how your days tend to flow.

- Do you have more free time in the morning, or are evenings better?

- Does your baby tend to take at least one decent nap during the day?

- If not, is your partner home at a reasonable hour and able to take over baby duties?

Figure out when you can have some time for yourself, then write it into your schedule, set reminders and do whatever you need to create the habit of consistent self-care.

You may be in a very busy season of life where these practices seem like an indulgence, but I assure you, they're not. In fact, those are the times when self-care becomes even more important. It's helpful to anticipate that life will, at times, get in the way of your plans. Just do what you can and pray the stars align more often than not. And remember, you may need to make sacrifices – be it accepting piles of laundry or cancelling non-essential obligations – so that you don't end up sacrificing yourself.

TIPS FOR FITTING SELF-CARE INTO YOUR LIFE WITH A BABY

When your baby sleeps

Perhaps the most convenient time to care for yourself is when your baby is sleeping. This may be during day naps or in the evening. If sleep is what you most need, then snooze when they do. This is especially important in the evening, as it will allow you to get as much deep and restorative rest as possible. If you find yourself not needing a day nap, you may have a few decent blocks of time to engage in other self-care activities. If your baby doesn't nap independently, try putting them in a baby carrier. This may allow you to do a little food prep, such as chopping vegetables, or tidying. You can also read a book or watch a show while holding your sleeping baby – just plan ahead so you have whatever you need close by.

If you need to work while your baby is sleeping, at least try to do something for yourself before sitting down at your desk. Make yourself a cup of tea and have a quick stretch, for example. This may not be your ideal form of self-care, but approaching whatever it is you can do with a nurturing mindset can help you to feel rejuvenated all the same.

Care for yourself while caring for your baby

Your baby needn't be sleeping for you to nurture yourself – you can engage in many self-care practices while they are awake. If they are happy being by themselves on a mat or in a bouncer, take that time to stretch, eat, cook or read.

Sometimes I make a game out of stretching by leaning towards Walt while he is lying on a rug – back and forth, back and forth, before coming in for a tickle. If your baby wants to be in your arms, you may be able to use a baby carrier and go for a walk.

For a more structured form of movement, seek out a mum and baby exercise class, where you can incorporate your bub into your workout or have them play with other babies. Group class gives you the added bonus of social connection, and you will also benefit from having your movements monitored by a qualified instructor who can ensure you're aiding, not hindering, your recovery. If you're not into exercise classes, playdates and local playgroups are a great way to socialise.

Other simple things you can do together, which will benefit you both, include getting outside in nature, having a bath and listening to music. All of these things have the ability to soothe fussiness and positively influence mood.

When your baby is a little older and starts eating, you can eat alongside them – that way you won't forget to nourish yourself. You may also be able to start doing more activities that are enjoyable for you both. I recall being thrilled when Joan reached the age where she was interested in drawing. To this day, when one (or both) of us needs a moment of calm, I bring out paper and pencils. Studies show colouring to be a meditative act, activating alpha brainwaves and helping us relax. As you can see, there are many things you can do with your baby and child that can also fill up your cup.

Enlist help from loved ones

If you're struggling to fit self-care into your day, ask your partner, family or friends to lend a hand. Remember, it won't always be this way, it's simply the nature of the season you're in. If you have people in your life who can, and want to, give you this kind of support, reach out to them. In the early days, when visitors pop by, don't feel obliged to sit and entertain them (unless spending time with said visitor is indeed the best way to replenish yourself). If you and your baby feel comfortable having a momentary change of hands, take that time for yourself.

You may like to schedule a weekly date when certain individuals stop by to help. My father visits us for 2 hours every Wednesday afternoon, and has done since Joan was a few months old. The knowledge that he was coming, and that I would be able to use that time to take a shower, prepare dinner or write, helped me get through the day (and the day leading up

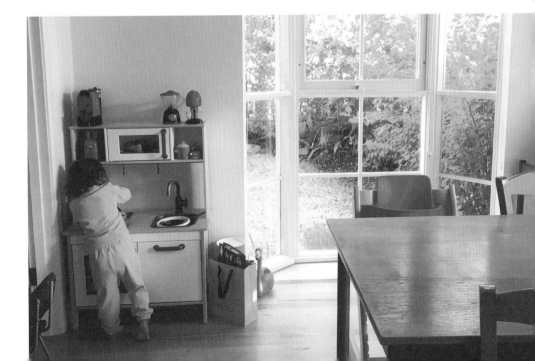

to it!). Think about who you might be able to call if you find yourself depleted; or, better yet, to help avoid depleting yourself in the first place. If you don't have a partner, family member, friend or neighbour who can provide this kind of support, you may want to think about hiring a trusted professional. You may only require their help every now and then, such as if you come down with mastitis, but it's important to know they're there should you need support.

Get started first thing

If you can, try to fit some self-care into your day as soon as you wake. Rather than reaching for your phone and tuning out (as many of us do), focus on tuning in to your body and mind. You might like to do a quick mindfulness exercise, stretch your body, listen to a favourite song, take a shower, write in your journal, step outside for some fresh air, read a few pages of a book or prepare a nourishing breakfast.

You certainly won't be able to do all of these things – in fact, you'll often be woken up by a screaming baby and may struggle to do anything for yourself. The point is to try to start your day by actively filling up your wellbeing cup in whatever way you can.

Care for yourself while your baby naps in the car (and read about your child's development)

Both my babies hated the car when they were young and would spend most rides screaming. Many babies do, however, enjoy being in the car and might fall asleep soon after the engine starts. This means you may find yourself parked at your destination for some time, waiting for them to wake up. If this happens, try to use the time for self-care. Plan ahead before you leave home to ensure you have a snack, a drink and some hand cream, plus a podcast to listen to, a book to read and/or your journal to write in. If you find yourself with none of these things, consider doing a mindfulness exercise (such as the one listed on page 14).

When Joan finally stopped screaming in the car and started having naps, I would use the time after I had parked to read about her development. Educating myself about the ways her brain and body were growing, the sort of challenges she may be experiencing, the behaviours I could expect from her and how to be supportive as she went through each developmental stage was actually a fantastic form of self-care for me.

Toddler behaviour can be really challenging, and it's easy to feel frustrated and impatient, especially if you're tired. Reading certain books (which I have listed on page 311) gave me guidance as to why she might be sharing big emotions or testing the boundaries I had put in place, and the types of phrases I could use when she did so that I could continue being the compassionate and consistent parent I always strive to be.

I still get frustrated at times, particularly now I have another baby who is waking me at night, but, as those books reminded me, that's ok. I don't hold my children or myself to impossibly high standards, and I'm not afraid to say sorry for losing my cool. Actually, I believe it's important they see me work through my emotions in a healthy way and offer myself compassion. It might just help them do the same as they move through their lives.

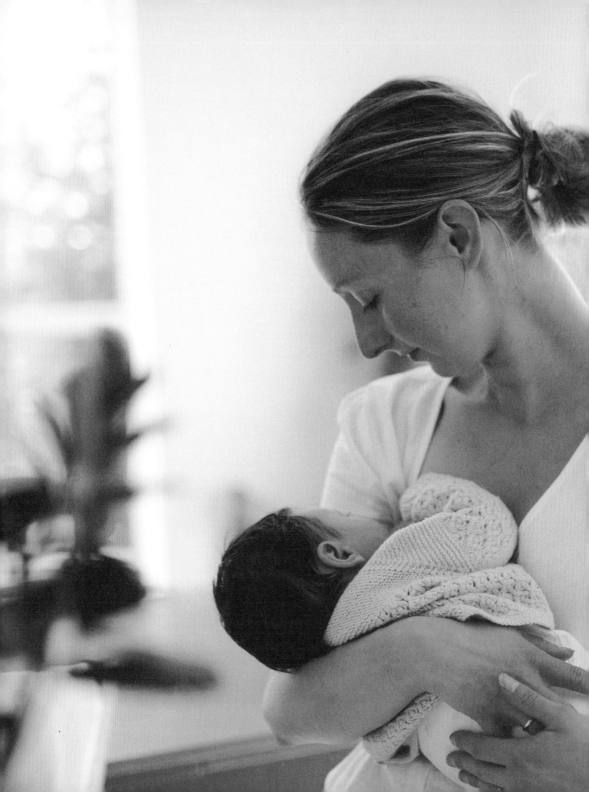

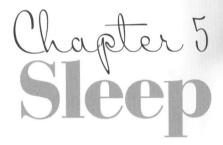

Chapter 5
Sleep

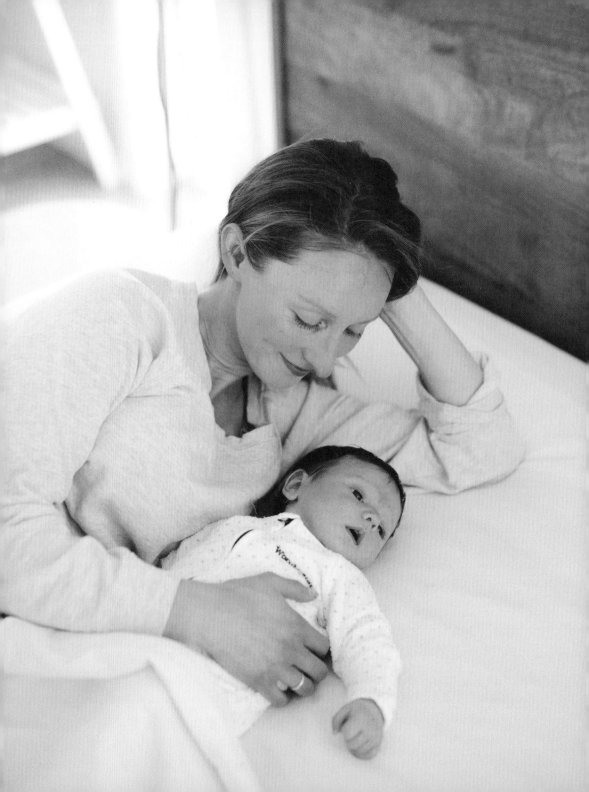

When Joan was very young, I remember thinking there was something I needed to be doing – some trick that I wasn't currently performing properly, that would allow her to sleep independently. I assumed that after I mastered this elusive technique she would sleep for long blocks all by herself, and my husband and I wouldn't have to deal with night waking any more.

My daughter was a wakeful baby, you see. Not what you would call an easy sleeper. As she was unable to fall asleep peacefully on her own, I would find myself doing all the things I had been cautioned against to help her sleep – I would hold her, rock her and feed her to sleep (sometimes all at once). Her bassinet went unused during the day, as did her pram. The only way I could get her to stay asleep was to keep her snug against my chest in the baby carrier or hold her in my arms. At night, I could (mercifully) get her to sleep in the bassinet for a solid 2–3-hour block (sometimes two blocks!), but after that she was done – no more bassinet, thanks, Mum.

By the time Joan was 4 months old, I couldn't get her to sleep away from me at all, not even for that first block at night. We tried moving her to her beautiful new cot, but that didn't work. In the end, I think she slept for a total of 2 hours in her cot (10 minutes here, 15 minutes there), which is less time than I spent looking into it online.

Despite trying all the tricks I'll discuss in this chapter, which can indeed encourage an independent sleeper, she wanted to be close to me (insisted on it, rather) and slept better when she was. And yet I continued to think I shouldn't let her. One evening, after a bizarre attempt to dangle my bare chest acrobatically over her cot in the hope that she would have a quick feed and fall back to sleep, I made a decision. I decided to stop focusing on what I thought I should be doing, and give myself permission to do what felt right to me as her mother.

Soon after the 'hovering over the cot' incident, I was talking to a girlfriend. This friend has two children who have slept fairly independently from a young age – 'good' sleepers, you might say. As I was discussing our challenges with sleep, my friend said something that helped me further embrace my situation. She told me that her children, who were 2 and 4 years old, didn't always sleep through the night; and that, more often than not, she is called into one of their rooms in the early hours for a cuddle.

It may seem silly to some (of course kids sometimes wake – adults do, too!), but this really changed things for me. I didn't realise how deeply I had internalised the rhetoric that there were babies who were 'good' sleepers who didn't wake and slept by themselves, and babies who were 'bad' sleepers who woke and needed assistance; and that once you taught the bad sleepers how to be good, all would be fixed. It's easy to see how new parents, who are unaware of normal infant sleep behaviour (as I was) and are perhaps a little sleep deprived and sensitive (like I was), can develop these beliefs.

When it comes to babies, there is so much talk about sleep – from whether your baby is sleeping through the night yet, to how long they take to fall asleep. These questions come from a good place. After all, sleep is crucial to our wellbeing.

How much we are (or aren't) sleeping can significantly influence our physical and mental health, as well as our overall sense of contentment as parents; and the reality is that many parents don't receive the support they require in order to survive the baby season without depleting themselves. Parents may also find themselves facing demanding and inflexible obligations (work or otherwise) in addition to caring for their baby, which makes ongoing sleep disruption even more calamitous.

Nevertheless, all the questions, advice and rules parents are inundated with about sleep can cause us to fret about our baby's perfectly normal behaviour, and lead us to act against our intuition. Sleep disruption is hard enough without that added stress and internal conflict. Knowing what is normal and having realistic expectations allows us to more easily give our baby and ourselves the acceptance, compassion and support required in order to get through this truly exhausting season.

Normal baby sleep behaviour

Babies have a pleasant life in utero. While tucked inside your womb, they are warm, comfortable, receive a steady supply of nourishment, and are soothed by the sounds and rhythmic rocking of your body. Birth brings babies out of this cosy den, exposing them to a flurry of new and overwhelming sensations, after which they continue to depend on you for protection, warmth, comfort, nourishment and help falling asleep.

Going into motherhood, I thought babies just slept when they were tired in whatever bed you placed them – 'Sweet dreams, see you later' sort of stuff. As it turns out, it doesn't tend to work that way. In order to fall asleep, babies need to feel relaxed and safe. And in order to feel this way, they generally require the assistance of their mother or other carer.

In our present parenting culture, however, we are cautioned against offering assistance. Instead, we are encouraged to teach our babies to fall asleep on their own and to soothe themselves back to sleep when they wake. I understand why we are given this advice, as caring for a wakeful baby who depends on you to help them sleep is utterly exhausting. Nevertheless, we tend to expect our babies to be able to sleep unassisted, and for long periods, before they can biologically, or are even supposed to.

Newborn babies haven't yet developed a circadian rhythm, meaning it doesn't matter if it's day or night, they will simply nap in blocks – 4 hours here, 2 hours there, and sometimes even less. A baby's stomach at birth is tiny, so they need to feed regularly. Thus, in the early days (and nights), it can feel like all you're doing is feeding your baby then helping them to sleep, while the moments you have to yourself to rest, shower and eat are few and far between, particularly if you need to pump breastmilk or if your baby doesn't sleep contentedly away from you.

As taxing as caring for a newborn can be, it's helpful to remember that your baby isn't manipulating you with their 'needy' behaviour (despite what you may hear); they are simply doing what they are meant to be doing in order to ensure their survival. You see, the comfort and milk you give your baby when they cry for you does so much more than stop their tears and fill their belly. Mother–baby contact helps to produce oxytocin, the hormone that encourages bonding and breastmilk production, and reduces stress levels in both mother and baby. When placed skin-to-skin with her baby, a mother will naturally adjust her body temperature in order to regulate that of her newborn baby. Babies also show more regulated, steady breathing when they are in close proximity to their mother or other adult carer. This phenomenon, called 'mutual regulation', is why experts recommend that babies sleep in the same room as parents, day and night, for at least the first 6–12 months of their life, when the risk of sudden infant death syndrome (SIDS), or sudden unexpected death in infancy (SUDI), is highest. It stands to reason, then, that we wouldn't want to override our baby's natural instinct to be close to their mother.

We also shouldn't necessarily want our baby to sleep through the night, which sounds crazy, I know, but hear me out. Night waking, at least when they're very young, can actually be beneficial. In the first 2 years of life, babies go through many stages of rapid and significant physical and cognitive growth. When they are experiencing these leaps, they need more nourishment and nurturing than usual, and not just during the day. Therefore, it's a good idea to release the expectation that night-time is just for sleep, especially when they are young.

Mothers who breastfeed release higher amounts of prolactin (the hormone responsible for milk production) overnight. This means that when babies wake to feed, they are helping to establish the correct milk supply for their needs. Night-time breastmilk also has higher levels of tryptophan, which promotes serotonin synthesis (known as the 'happy hormone') and encourages healthy brain development. It also promotes the production of melatonin, the hormone that helps us sleep and aids the development of your baby's circadian rhythm. Breastmilk-related benefits aside, your baby's night waking can also be an innate, protective mechanism that ensures they keep breathing.

This is not to say that babies who naturally sleep for long stretches are necessarily putting themselves at risk, or that their mothers aren't producing wonderful milk – rather, I say this to reassure you that night waking is normal and that the contact and care you give them at 2 am does a lot of good. Whether you offer them the breast, bottle or a loving touch, you are helping your baby to feel secure and fostering resilience while their brain rapidly develops, which will actually help them to sleep well in the long term. It can be helpful to remind yourself of this when your baby continues to wake overnight, or when they go from sleeping through to once again being wakeful – both of which are common and will probably happen.

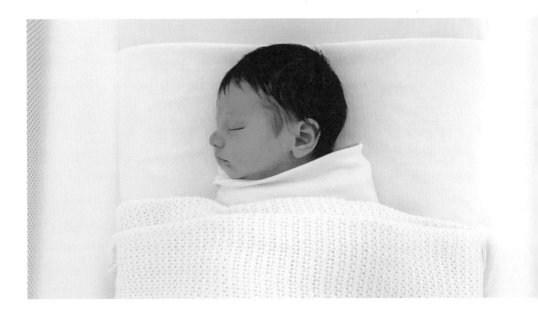

When your baby is 3 months old, you may find things begin to shift. It is around this age that babies develop a circadian rhythm, meaning they can tell the difference between night and day. As a result, they start sleeping less during the day and more at night. You can help encourage this pattern by exposing them to lots of natural light during the day, and dimming the lights and avoiding bright screens in the evenings (for night wakings, I use a salt lamp, as it has a gentle, womb-like glow and also makes it easier for me to fall back to sleep).

In addition, your older baby will have a bigger stomach that can hold more milk, which means they may not need to feed quite so often from a hunger perspective (though they may want to feed for comfort and connection). All of this might translate to longer blocks of sleep overnight, which means you, too, might be sleeping more.

I vividly remember the first time Joan gave me an uninterrupted, 3-hour block of sleep – I felt completely revived. Gradually, these longer blocks became more frequent and predictable. We'd start off with 2, 3 (sometimes even 4!) hours of sleep at the start of the night, before she'd wake for a feed and go down for another decent snooze.

The time spent feeding and burping was getting shorter, too, which meant I was awake less overall. 'Ok,' I thought. 'This is how it'll be for a while until she eventually starts sleeping through.' A few weeks later, though, everything changed. Suddenly, Joan was too interested in the world to feed for long periods during the day. She preferred to feed at night, which was also when her brain was processing the new information she was receiving during the day and practising new skills (such as rolling over and crawling). All of this translated to wakeful, restless nights and tired days.

Thankfully, not too long after I began frantically searching online for an explanation, a friend sent me an article by breastfeeding expert Pinky McKay, which reassured me that my daughter's behaviour was perfectly normal, and that the 4-month sleep 'regression' was actually a sign of cognitive 'progression' (though it certainly didn't feel that way when I was being woken every hour).

These sort of sleep regressions/progressions can happen at any stage, such as when babies are sick or teething, or going through developmental leaps (4 months is a common age, as is 8–10 months, when babies begin to develop separation anxiety). It can also happen when they're experiencing change in their everyday life, such as moving house, starting daycare or the birth of a sibling. Indeed, night waking is extremely common. It's inconvenient and challenging, but common and understandable.

It's baffling, then, that so much emphasis is placed on getting your baby to sleep through the night, when research shows it is simply not a realistic goal when they're young. No matter how you define 'sleeping through the night' (some refer to this as a 5–8 hour stretch, whereas others take it to mean 7 pm to 7 am), most babies are unable to do so until they are closer to 1 year old (often 2!), and even then it may not happen consistently. I share this information not to make you feel as though the sleep thing is hopeless. Some babies do actually sleep for long periods fairly independently and consistently, and there are things you can do to encourage this (see page 134). Others don't, however, and won't for some time, and it's helpful to know that this is normal – expected, even.

Even when you know a certain behaviour is normal, you will surely still find yourself questioning, worrying and searching the internet, which is why I have provided some resources for you on page 311. Refer to them for reassurance and to remind yourself that in order to care for your baby day and night, you also need to care for yourself. While it's normal to feel tired as a new parent, if you are struggling and not feeling like yourself, it's important to seek assistance from your village and/or an empathetic health care provider. Babies require selfless care, it's true, but as the saying goes, you cannot pour from an empty cup.

Tune in to your family's needs

Babies are wired to wake regularly for nourishment and comfort, and their needs must be respected. Yet we must also recognise and respect the impact this has on the wellbeing of parents. Ongoing sleep disruption is no joke, and studies suggest we all differ in our capacity to tolerate it. We also have different circumstances that impact our ability to surrender to our baby's sleep needs, including our mental health status, work commitments and whether we have a supportive partner who can help share the load. Thus, when deciding on your family's sleeping arrangement, you will need to take into consideration the needs of each family member. Parents won't always need to be hyper-vigilant about getting as much sleep as possible, but during the season of sleep disruption it needs to be a priority.

Ideally, both parents will be able to help out with night care. If, however, you are struggling with a postnatal mood disorder, you may need to prioritise your sleep and have your partner step up. Similarly, if you have a partner who works outside the home in a job that requires they be well rested (as a taxi driver or surgeon, for example), you may need to make the bulk of the sleep sacrifices. If both you and your partner are working, you may decide to take turns for half the night or have one parent be in charge on certain nights of the week. If you are a single parent or don't have a supportive partner, you will need to rely more heavily on your village for support and catch up on sleep whenever you can. You will also want to get to bed as soon as possible at night. The same goes for mothers who are caring for more than one baby – be it twins, triplets or babies close in age.

Finally, consider where each of your family members might sleep. As it is recommended that babies sleep in the same room as their caregiver for at least the first 6 months, you may wish to place a bassinet beside your bed or use a co-sleeper attachment, which allows your baby to lie next to you without being in your bed. When your baby reaches a certain age, they may prefer to sleep more independently, and will do better in their own room. If this isn't the case, your partner, depending on their work demands, may want to sleep in a separate room on occasion to avoid being woken.

Or it may be that your baby rests better when sleeping in your bed. Should you choose to bed-share, it is crucial you are aware of the risks involved, as SIDS/SUDI guidelines recommend that you do not share a sleeping surface with your baby (see pages 142–3 for more information).

Beyond the safety concerns about bed-sharing, some parents are hesitant to do so for fear that their baby will never sleep on their own. Keep in perspective that bed-sharing with your baby when they're young doesn't mean they will still be bed-sharing as teenagers (although, if they feel comfortable enough to come into your room for a midnight cuddle when they're 14 and experiencing a whole new set of overwhelming cognitive changes, that is a good thing).

Try to keep an open mind when deciding on sleeping arrangements. It may very well not work out as you had imagined when setting up your baby's nursery, and that's ok. The goal is to ensure you are all as healthy, rested and content as possible.

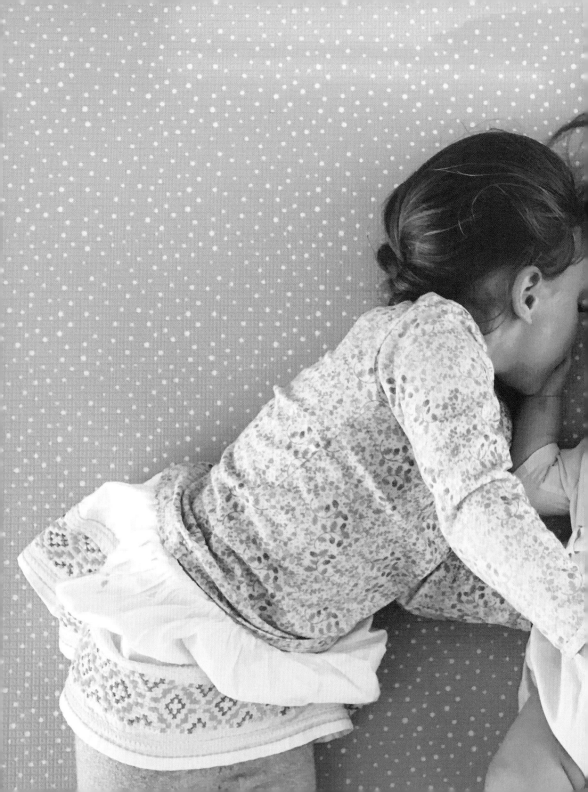

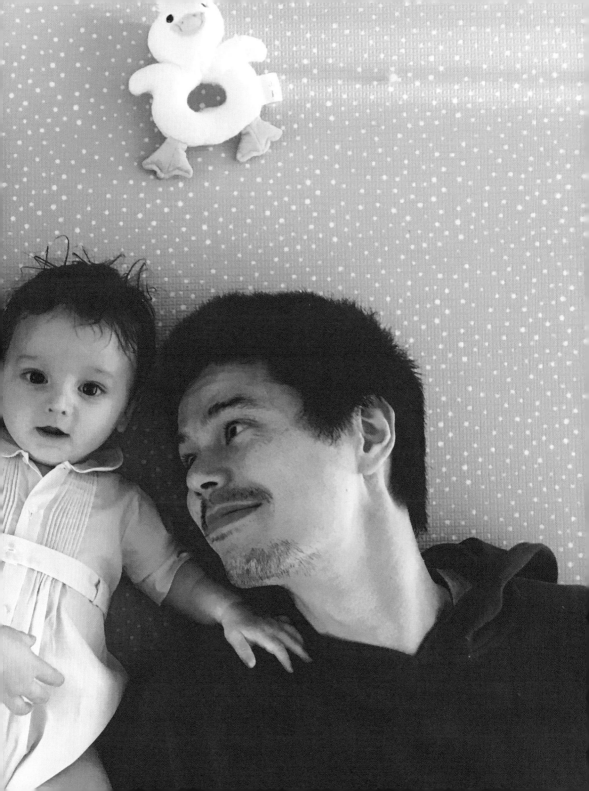

Helping babies sleep peacefully

We've established that most babies need help falling asleep, and that they often wake and require assistance falling back to sleep. On the following pages are some suggestions on how to provide this assistance, but remember: every baby has a unique nature and set of needs, which can change as they grow. That is to say that these ideas may or may not work for you, or they may work initially and then stop working (or vice versa). The best thing you can do is tune in to your baby's needs, seek support when you require it and advice when you want it, and, ultimately, do what feels right. If it stops feeling right or their (or your) needs change, you can always do something else.

THE NEWBORN DAYS

An effective way to help your newborn baby fall asleep is to replicate the sensations of the womb. This means ensuring they are warm and snug, with a belly full of milk (make sure they've had the chance to burp up any wind). Ask your midwife or a friend to show you how to swaddle your baby, as this tends to help them sleep contentedly for longer periods. Music or background noise can be helpful, whether you sing a lullaby, make 'shhh' noises or use white noise (more on this below). You may like to rock them to sleep with gentle, rhythmic motions and perhaps give them something to suck on – whether it's your nipple, a bottle or a dummy. Yes, it's ok to feed your baby to sleep, despite what you may hear. You may possibly be setting them up to want this comfort every time they sleep, but if it works for them (and you) and allows them to sleep peacefully, don't hesitate to do this, especially while they are young. Some babies happily drift off without this song and dance, but the majority require some assistance, particularly if you miss their early tired cues and they get overtired.

Contrary to what you may think, when babies are very tired it's actually more difficult for them to fall asleep. Part of getting to know your baby – what their cries mean, how they like to be fed and held – will therefore involve getting to know their tired cues. Yawning and rubbing eyes are two of the more obvious signs that it's time to get your baby ready for a nap, but their cues can certainly be more subtle. When Joan was a baby, I came to understand that if she was staring off into the distance in a daze, she needed to sleep. Walt, on the other hand, becomes red around the eyes. Look out for those tired cues and, when you recognise them, make sure your baby is warm, dry, comfortable and full. You will then want to put them down while they are drowsy but awake, so they can fall asleep on their own …

I know, I know! To those who have babies, this commonly given advice might seem preposterous. One blog reader told me that upon hearing it, 'I cackled like a maniac, partly because I was so tired but I also genuinely thought it was a joke.' The thing is, though, it's actually good advice, as a baby who learns to fall asleep on their own will be a much easier sleeper. What those words should be swiftly followed with is the statement that most babies won't be able to do this right away, and many won't for a long time. That doesn't mean you can't keep gently trying; just don't be disheartened when they continue to need assistance. It won't always be like this – even if you never actively teach a baby to fall asleep on their own and soothe themselves back to sleep, they all eventually learn how to do so. While you wait for them to get there, one of the most important things you can do is ensure they feel safe and loved.

TIPS FOR ENCOURAGING AN INDEPENDENT SLEEPER

If you wish to transition away from assisting your baby to sleep as described above (as many parents like to do once they pass the newborn days), there are a number of things you can do to encourage your baby to sleep independently. It's important to know, though, that the gentle tips that follow will not teach your child to sleep this way if they are not ready to do so. In other words, they won't force the independence issue. Rather, they will help you to create the conditions whereby your baby may learn to sleep independently if they are ready.

Even if after trying these suggestions, your baby remains wakeful and dependent (as my first baby did), remind yourself that it can take time before they get the hang of this sleep thing, no matter how consistent you are. At the very least, these tips should help make sleep a more pleasant experience for both of you. Don't forget that if your baby is going through a developmental leap, all bets are off and you may need to wait until it passes before they respond to these methods (or any others you may try).

Bed routine

What you do in the lead-up to sleep doesn't matter so much in the early weeks, but once your baby begins to develop their circadian rhythm, an evening bedtime routine can help them switch over to night sleep mode. **Note:** You can do this routine for day sleeps too, if it works for you.

A simple night-time routine might look like this: make sure their belly is full and they have burped if they need to; dim the lights; and ensure they are comfortable and relaxed. A warm bath is nice to do before bed, and afterwards, if your baby is agreeable, you may like to give them a gentle massage before getting them into their pyjamas. Lavender essential oil is commonly used to help encourage relaxation and sleep, though it's absolutely vital you seek advice to ensure you are using essential oils safely – such as diluting them considerably, never applying directly to your baby's skin and not using them on young babies.

You may like to read your baby a book and/or sing a lullaby. Choose a song that represents bedtime, which they can carry with them throughout their childhood as their goodnight tune. In my family, we have a little saying – 'niney poppins, in the morney see' – which my grandmother said to my mother as a child, which my mother said to me, and which I now say to my children. Joan often says it to her toys before bed, though she has modified it slightly, saying, 'Mary Poppins, see you in the morning.'

During winter, you can warm your baby's bed with a hot water bottle, removing it before your baby is laid down. This can help make bed more inviting. A cosy swaddle or baby sleeping bag (depending on where they're at developmentally), might help too.

All of these little rituals help your baby to know it's time to slow down and rest. They may also allow them to drift off to sleep without being fed or rocked – you just have to see how they go and trust that they'll get there when they're ready. Remember, every baby is different.

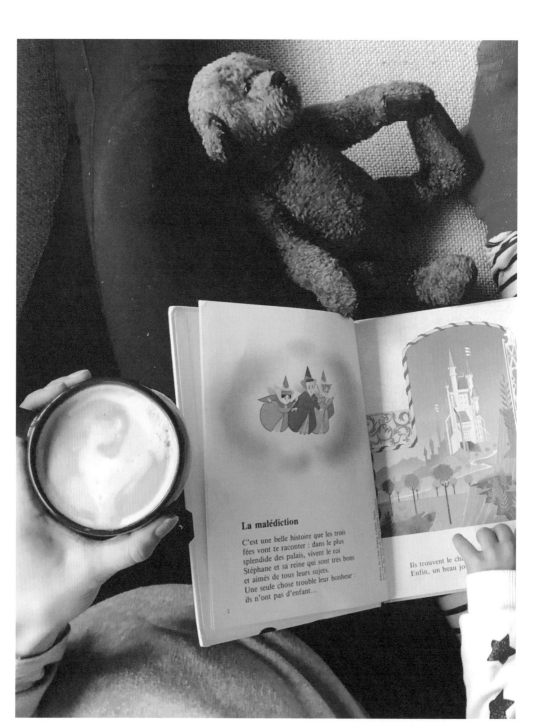

La malédiction

C'est une belle histoire que les trois
fées vont te raconter : dans le plus
splendide des palais, vivent le roi
Stéphane et sa reine qui sont très bons
et aimés de tous leurs sujets.
Une seule chose trouble leur bonheur :
ils n'ont pas d'enfant...

2

Ils trouvent le cha
Enfin, un beau jo

Comforter

A comforter is a specific toy or blanket that comforts your baby and helps them fall asleep. The idea is you bring the chosen comforter into your baby's sleep environment early on, to help them develop this association. You may like to place the comforter between you and your baby while they are being fed or rocked to sleep (that way it will end up smelling like you, which is your baby's favourite scent). There are lots of options on the market that are designed for this purpose. If you do find a comforter that works for your baby, you may like to get two, in case you end up losing one or need to wash it. Be sure to follow guidelines to make sure whatever you are using is safe.

Dummy

If a parent doesn't wish to feed their baby to sleep, they may like to offer their child a dummy (also known as a pacifier or soother) in bed. Not only can a dummy help soothe your baby back to sleep when they rouse (the sucking action helps comfort them), dummies have been shown to reduce their risk of SIDS/SUDI. Just be aware that your baby may wake in the night if their dummy has fallen out of their mouth and require help putting it back in. You may eventually have to wean them off the dummy, but I'd pop that firmly in the 'deal with it later' basket. Dentists and orthodontists have opinions on the style of dummy you may wish to use (and whether a dummy is better than a thumb), so look into it, ask questions and decide what you are comfortable with. Joan refused a dummy, despite multiple attempts with multiple styles. In the end, I suppose I became her dummy, as she would breastfeed back to sleep whenever she woke. Do what works for you.

White noise

Babies are used to hearing loud, muffled noise in the womb. To replicate this sound you can use a white noise machine, a fan or an app on your phone to help them to drift off to sleep. Make sure whatever you are using isn't placed close to their head or turned up too loud (certainly not louder than their crying). Also be sure to switch your phone to airplane mode before placing it near their bed.

Temperature

The temperature of the room in which your baby is sleeping is another thing to consider. Studies show people sleep better in cooler environments, so make sure they are wearing weather-appropriate pyjamas made of breathable fabrics, and don't overload them with blankets. On the other hand, you don't want them to be too cold. It can take a bit of trial and error before you figure out what arrangement works best for your baby. If they constantly kick off their blankets then cry out because they're chilly, you might like to place them in a baby sleeping bag (one designed specifically for babies to sleep in). On warm nights, a fan can help circulate air around the room, while doubling as a white noise machine.

Sleep during the day

If your baby has napped well throughout the day (meaning they're not overtired) and haven't stayed awake for too long before bed, there's a better chance they will fall asleep easily and be less wakeful overnight. As they say, sleep begets sleep. To ensure your baby is well rested, you may like to stick to a schedule during the day or go with the flow and follow their tired cues – this is a personal choice.

Other ideas

There are presently some really neat contraptions on the market that can help your baby sleep independently and for long periods, by helping to soothe them to sleep when it's bedtime, and soothing them back to sleep when they rouse. Bassinets that rock and mechanical dolls that 'breathe' are just some examples. Obviously this isn't teaching them to sleep on their own, but as I have said, it can take some time before babies are capable of doing this. And if this helps you to get rest in the meantime (and if you can afford it), then why not?

Having tried these suggestions, don't worry if you end up wearing your baby in a sling for every nap (like I did), or continue rocking and feeding your baby to sleep (like I did) far beyond those newborn months. Yes, your baby will generally call out for you if they have fallen asleep in your arms or on the breast, and suddenly wake up alone in a bed. But if you are happy to keep assisting them and soothing them back to sleep, it's perfectly fine to remain your baby's sleep association.

Allowing your child to be dependent for a period does not mean they will be dependent forever. In fact, it means quite the opposite. Be sure to look out for signs that they are ready to settle on their own, though, so you don't continue assisting them unnecessarily. When I sensed it was time for Joan to move away from napping in the baby carrier, we transitioned to napping in a bed – very gradually shifting from wearing, rocking and feeding her to sleep, to simply lying down next to her and feeding her to sleep. When we weaned, I replaced the feeding with other things, like cuddling and storytelling.

A note on sleep training

When Joan was 5 months old, I met a friend and her baby for a playdate, during which she told me she had started sleep training her baby. In sharing her experience, my friend told me she had taken her daughter (who was perhaps 7 months old at the time) to sleep school, in the hope she would stop waking overnight. And it worked! Until she got sick, that is. Or was teething, travelling or going through one of the many developmental leaps babies do when they're little. When this happened, my friend told me her daughter would revert to being wakeful and she would need to train her baby all over again. Admittedly, this retraining period didn't take as long as the first time, but even so, to me it all seemed like so much work.

Having just experienced the 4-month sleep regression with Joan, I thought to myself, 'When are babies not going through some sort of experience that leaves them prone to wakefulness?' Sleep training is a contentious topic in the parenting world. Mothers readily feel judged for their decision to train or not to train. And yet no mother can know precisely what another is experiencing. Our lives are complex and circumstances unique, and many parents feel sleep training is the best option for their family. Through attending sleep school or having a consultant come to their home, they may gain valuable insights regarding their child's tired cues and how to create a routine that allows their child to sleep peacefully.

On the other hand, some parents feel pressure to train their child because they have been told that their baby should be sleeping through the night, and that the way they are responding to their child's needs is stopping them from doing so. Yet as I have mentioned above, it's entirely normal for your baby not to sleep through the night, and to wake in search of comfort.

When deciding how you want to tackle the sleep thing, you need to, once again, look to your intuition and honour the needs of your entire family unit. Your baby needs to feel secure and loved in order to grow into a healthy and happy person, and you need to be getting at least some rest in order to be a healthy and happy parent. If you do decide to go down the sleep training path, it's important you seek advice from sensitive, qualified professionals who appreciate that every child and family is different, who respect your baby's need for comfort and who don't simply tell you to leave your baby to cry alone in a room all night without responding. As a mother, you should always be encouraged to listen to your intuition. There are numerous ways to teach your baby to sleep independently for long periods – some gently nudging, others forcing it long before the child is ready. I would encourage you to be gentle.

I mentioned my friend, and ventured ever so slightly into the testy topic of sleep training, not just to encourage you to do what feels right for your family, but to illustrate how I came to know what was best for mine. Hearing this mothers' (and other's) experience, helped me to recognise that I didn't want to train my child to sleep independently or self-soothe before she was ready. In my case, it felt so much better, and seemed a heck of a lot easier, to surrender to the fact that my daughter wanted to be close to me. As it turns out, that was the 'trick' that finally allowed us all to sleep soundly.

Our story of bed-sharing

Our family ended up bed-sharing for 18 months. Bed-sharing, when your baby is actually in bed with you, is different from co-sleeping, which refers to your baby sleeping in the same room as you (whether that's in a bassinet, cot or a co-sleeper attached to the side of your bed). Before I share our experience, I want to outline some safe bed-sharing tips.

Safe bed-sharing

Bed-sharing can be extremely hazardous, and may cause infant death. The following must be considered:

- Do not bed-share with premature or low-birth-weight babies.

- Do not bed-share if you are a smoker, have been drinking alcohol or are on medication that alters your ability to be aware of your sleeping baby.

- Research shows us that mothers are especially attuned to their baby's needs, even when they're sleeping (meaning when your baby rouses, so will you); this, however, isn't the case with your partner or older children. If your partner is a deep sleeper, they should sleep in another bed. If your partner is sharing the bed, place your baby next to you, not between you and your partner.

- Older siblings should be in a separate bed away from your baby.

- Ensure your mattress is very firm. Do not sleep with your baby on a couch, waterbed, hammock or beanbag.

- Place your baby to sleep on their back.

- Do not swaddle your baby if you are bed-sharing. They need to be able to move their arms to help them reposition their head, if required.

- Keep your bedding minimal. There should be no pillows near your baby and no loose blankets. A fitted sheet pulled up as far as your hips will do, and if it's winter, put your baby (and yourself) in warm pyjamas.

- Make sure there are no gaps between your bed and the headboard where baby's head could get trapped.

- If your baby is rolling, it's best to place your mattress low, on or near the floor, to avoid them rolling off the bed and hurting themselves.

See page 311 for a resource that provides additional tips on safe bed-sharing, including how to position your baby in relation to your body.

Even if you don't plan on bed-sharing, I encourage you to take a look. Research shows most parents are likely to end up bed-sharing with their baby at some point, and it's best to educate yourself ahead of time so you know how to do so safely.

I certainly didn't plan on bed-sharing with my babies. In fact, I remember discussing the topic with Ben when I was pregnant for the first time. I had just visited a girlfriend who told me her 15-month-old son, partner and herself all slept in the same bed. Later that night, Ben and I categorically agreed that we wouldn't bed-share. He feared he'd roll on top of the baby, whereas to me it just seemed unnecessary. Babies slept in cots, so why would you need them in your bed? Then my daughter was born, and I did a complete turnaround.

Buzzed after her birth, I stayed up most of the night holding her. When I grew tired I handed her to Ben so I could sleep. This was our routine every night for the first 2–3 weeks while he was on leave, and while it was clearly unsustainable, we didn't care because it felt right. Or at least, it was the happy medium between what we felt we should do, which was force her to sleep away from us in a bassinet against her will, and what we wanted to do, which was sleep alongside her. Eventually our daughter started accepting the bassinet at the start of the night, which allowed Ben and me to get more rest, but that didn't last long. And this back-and-forth between should we/shouldn't we bed-share continued.

In the beginning, I was mostly hesitant because of her size. Joan was quite small at birth, just 2.75 kg (6.1 lb) at 38 weeks. She felt tiny and fragile, and I wasn't confident in my ability to keep her safe. It wasn't until she was almost 3 months old that we stopped worrying about this. But we had other concerns. We worried that by allowing her to lie beside us, we would ruin her ability to sleep independently. As a parent, you want to make sure you're doing right by your baby, and we had been told that an independent sleeper was what we should have been aiming for. The other reason I was reluctant to bed-share was I didn't know how to do it. I was aware that some of my friends were sleeping with their babies, and that I had slept alongside my mother as a baby, but I hadn't discussed the details, such as where to put them.

Mothers have been bed-sharing with their babies for centuries and many cultures around the world continue to do so. In Australia and other Western societies, however, medical professionals don't endorse the practice and even caution parents against it. This is understandable, as there are definite safety concerns. Yet because many parents will find themselves bed-sharing with their baby, even if only briefly, we need to be taught how to do it safely so that we can minimise the risks.

Eventually, Ben and I were able to move past our concerns and educate ourselves as to how to keep our baby safe while sharing a bed. We splurged on a king-sized bed with a firm mattress and found that for the first time since Joan was born, we felt rested.

Bed-sharing isn't without its challenges, though. When we first brought Joan into our bed, I found myself hyper-attuned to her every move and unable to sleep deeply (though this lasted only a week or so). Joan was seemingly hyper-attuned to my presence, too (as she had been since birth), and would wake every time I tried to sneak off to watch a show with Ben or use the toilet. At one point I even kept a potty under our bed so I could wee while resting my hand on her belly (looking back that seems nuts, but hey, you do what you've got to do).

Bed-sharing didn't magically stop her from waking or wanting me, but it certainly helped her to wake less often, provided I remained close. And when she did wake, she would simply reach out for me – instantly falling back to sleep with a just touch or quick breastfeed. Ben and I were no longer battling to get her back into her bassinet or cot. In fact, I rarely had to get out of bed. It was great! I could be the mother she needed and the mother I wanted to be – providing her with comfort and nourishment through all her leaps and life experiences, with as little disruption to my sleep as possible.

Not everyone has a similar bed-sharing experience. Some parents find themselves doing it out of necessity, as it is the only way their baby will sleep contentedly, yet their own sleep may suffer. Their baby may kick and squirm all night, and one parent may remain resistant. Ben and I were lucky in that Joan wasn't a wriggler, and we wholeheartedly agreed bed-sharing was the right decision for our family.

I'm still bed-sharing, only now with Walt. As it turns out, he is quite similar to Joan in the sleep department. Both have wanted to sleep close to me (whether in the carrier or the bed) and sleep peacefully when they are; and both have woken fairly frequently in the night, returning straight back to sleep after some contact.

There are a few of differences second time around, though. For one, I haven't hesitated to offer Walt assistance to fall sleep. I freely hold him, rock him or feed him to sleep – whatever he needs. Also, Walt was bigger at birth, so he and I have bed-shared from the beginning, while Ben has

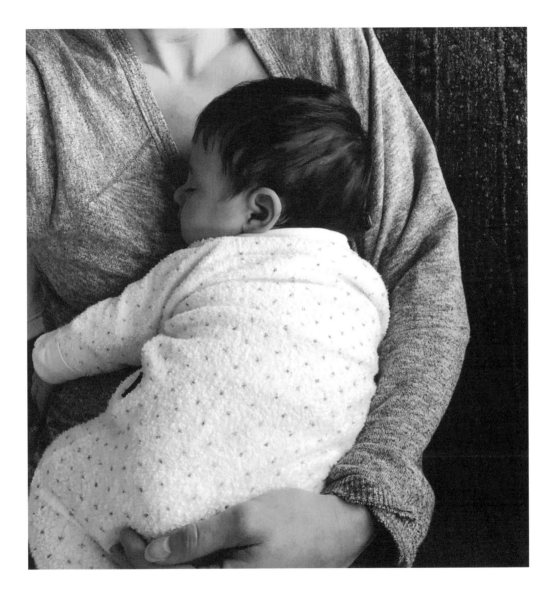

stayed with Joan in her room (to ensure he gets a good night's rest and also to be there for her when she needs him).

Lastly, it's not uncommon for Walt to fall asleep without assistance. This usually happens at night, after his evening feed with me, and a quick cuddle and chat with Ben – when Walt will, on occasion, look for me, close his eyes and drift off to sleep. The first time this happened (when he was 3 months old) I was dazzled, I assure you. Oh, and I can also leave the bed to use the toilet. I'm sure it helps that I'm more relaxed as a second-time mum. But mostly, it's just him. He's a different baby.

If you have been told that by assisting your baby to go to sleep you are creating a 'rod for your own back', know this: our ability as mothers to soothe our baby with our body is downright amazing, not to mention immensely beneficial to our baby's development. So if it feels good and right, I say go ahead and create that rod. With time, when your baby is ready, it might fall away on its own. And if it doesn't (and you no longer want, or are able, to keep it there), know that you can always remove it.

NIGHT WEANING

Bed-sharing and breastfeeding on demand worked wonderfully for us until Joan was 13 months old, when she began waking every hour for milk. While night waking is normal, and generally increases when your baby is going through a period of physical or cognitive growth, this behaviour continued for 2 months, at which stage I was utterly exhausted. And so I decided to replace the comfort of breastmilk with the comfort of a cuddle, in the hope it would encourage her to sleep for longer blocks.

Night weaning, or any sort of gentle sleep training, is never going to be fun, but the good thing about doing it when your child is older is that they have had time to develop a secure attachment. This means they're less likely to be distressed by the change (provided you continue to show them love and comfort) and more likely to just be, for want of a better term, pissed off.

Upon recommendation from a friend, we followed Dr Jay Gordon's night weaning protocol, which took us through different steps when our daughter woke – from rocking to cuddling. There was some grizzling, but it was minimal. She wasn't distressed. Eventually, Joan stopped waking every hour, and when she did wake (which was still a few times a night), she was content falling back to sleep snuggled in my arms.

TRANSITIONING TO HER OWN BED

Later on, when Joan was 18 months old, we moved her into her own bed, in her own room. While we still enjoyed bed-sharing, I intuitively felt it was time. We were hoping to have a second baby, and wanted Joan in her own room well before the end of my pregnancy. She was also waking less overnight at that stage, often just once, and I sensed she would do well with the transition. After speaking to Joan about the change, and seeing her enthusiasm at the thought of having her own bed, we decided to go ahead. The first week was one big sleepover. Joan and I went to bed together and got up together in the morning. She loved her bed (which was a single bed frame with the legs cut off, plus a bed rail to prevent her rolling out), and the two of us would play on it during the day, reading her toys a story before putting them to bed. After the initial week I continued to lie down with her while she drifted off, then I would get up and leave her to sleep on her own.

As you might recall, this had previously been impossible. Until about a month before we made the change, I couldn't leave her side without her waking. But she had recently become less wakeful and I could walk away with ease, often not hearing a peep out of her for 2–3 hours. Ben and I could once again sit down to eat dinner together and watch a movie away from sleeping Joan. Though I must say, neither of us minded the bed picnics we had when she was younger. To us, it was just a momentary change in our lifestyle, which felt so much better than trying to get her to sleep independently before she was ready (remember my cot acrobatics?). I guess that's why we kept it up for all those months. And I guess that's why Ben continues to squeeze alongside her when she wakes overnight.

Joan took well to the change but continued to wake most nights. She's now 3 and is still quite wakeful. I can count on one hand the number of times she has slept through from bedtime until after 5 am without calling out for us. But that's ok. I no longer expect her to sleep in the way I envisaged before becoming a mother. 'Sweet dreams, see you later' isn't our reality. Not yet at least.

Your sleep story might be different from mine. It probably will be. Nevertheless, I have shared mine as an antidote to all the sleep dos and don'ts you will hear as a new parent. Real-life stories remind you that every baby and every family is different, and hopefully leave you feeling empowered to listen to your intuition.

Your sleep

Sleep is crucial to our wellbeing, no matter what life stage we're in. Thanks to our modern lifestyle, many of us aren't getting enough. With the flick of a switch we can light up a room or turn on a screen, thereby disrupting our body's production of melatonin (the sleep hormone) and altering our natural circadian rhythm. Stress can also impact our body's ability to rest.

During pregnancy, it becomes even harder to get the sleep we need. Some women struggle with pregnancy-related insomnia and leg cramps, and many find themselves waking frequently to use the toilet. Getting comfortable can also be a challenge, especially in the final weeks. All of this is great training for the postnatal period, when our newborn baby continually disrupts our sleep. After birth, we may also experience hormonal changes that alter our ability to rest, or feel too attuned to our baby to switch off or sleep soundly. In short, most of us won't be getting the sleep we need during this time, which is why we need to maximise what we can get.

Give yourself the opportunity to rest

This means going to bed whenever you can throughout the day, and as soon as possible at night. During periods of extreme wakefulness, such as when your baby has a cold or is going through a developmental leap, this practice becomes particularly important and sleep should move to the top of your to-do list. Lie down during your baby's nap – even if you don't drift off, your body will benefit from the rest, particularly in the early days and weeks after childbirth.

Avoid bright lights

Exposure to bright lighting at night can impact your ability to sleep, so keep the lights low when it's dark outside. You may like to invest in some dimmer switches or a lamp that omits gentle, non-disruptive light, such as a salt lamp.

Minimise screens

Like bright lights, staring at a light-emitting screen (whether it's the TV, computer or phone) can make it harder get good sleep. Instead of looking at a screen, read a book or, at the very least, switch your phone or computer to night mode. Alternatively, you might consider purchasing glasses that block the blue light emitted by screens, which can alter melatonin production and hinder your ability to fall asleep.

Pillows and bedding

Getting comfortable at night can be tricky during pregnancy, especially if you're not used to lying on your side. Placing pillows around your body and between your legs can alleviate discomfort, while also helping with pelvic alignment. Make sure your bedding is not too heavy and causing you to overheat, as we tend to sleep better when we're not too hot.

Do for yourself as you do for your baby

Follow the tips on page 135 and create your own night-time ritual – take a bath, diffuse lavender oil, give yourself a massage or read a book. These relaxing practices are just as beneficial for adults.

Eat

Going for long periods without eating and/or not having balanced meals can cause dips in your blood sugar levels. This, in turn, can make it harder for you to fall asleep and leave you prone to wakefulness. A snack before bed that contains protein, fat and high-fibre carbohydrates (for example, a banana with nut butter) can do wonders.

Just be sure to avoid eating too close to bedtime, to minimise your chance of experiencing heartburn, and don't drink lots of liquid before you fall asleep (as you'll need to get up even more frequently to wee).

Move your body

Studies show that fitting in some form of exercise during the day helps you sleep better at night. It can also improve your energy levels after a poor night's sleep.

Journalling

If you struggle to switch off your mind at night, jotting down some of your thoughts before bed can help you to relax into sleep. You might like to end with a gratitude practice (see page 26–7) to help shift you into a positive mindset.

Chapter 6
Nourishing Yourself

PART 1

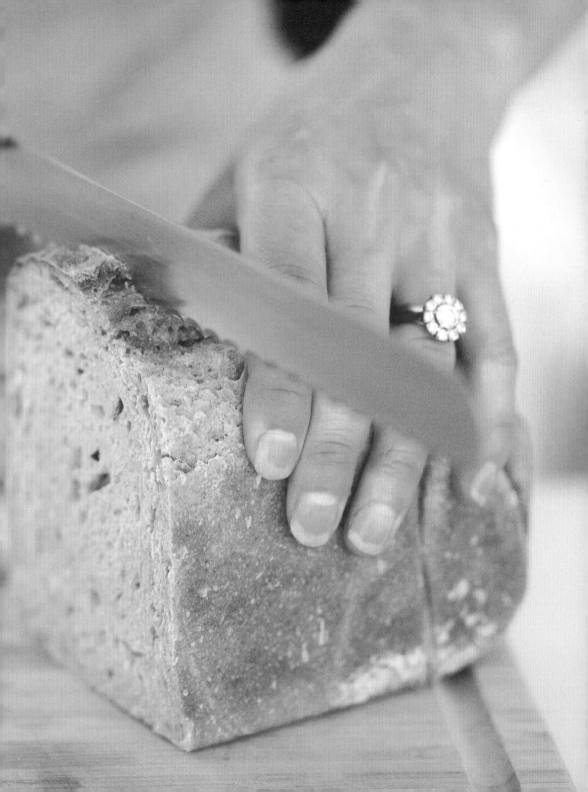

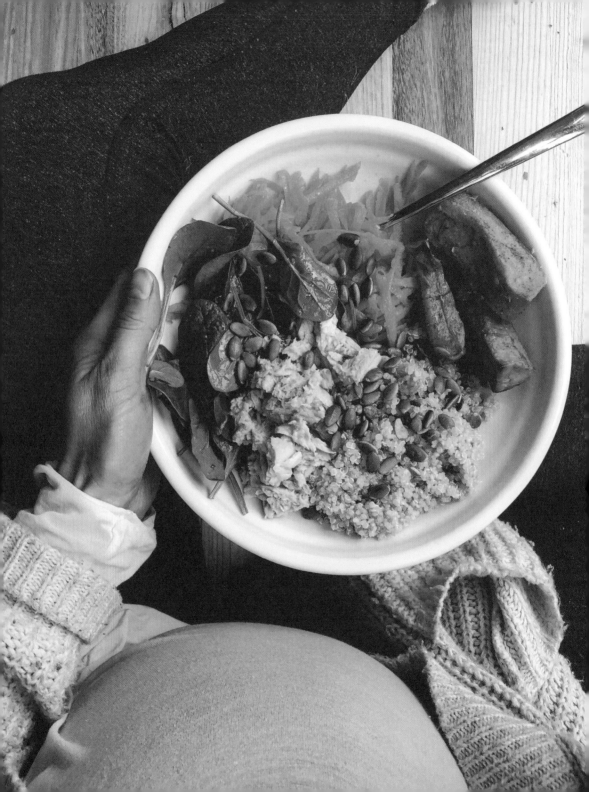

When a woman discovers she is pregnant, there is often a shift in the way she approaches food. She may feel compelled to eat with newfound intention, consuming as many vegetables as possible, 'for the baby'. Or she may relax restrictions that were previously in place, consuming as many doughnuts as possible, 'for the baby'. She may also experience food aversions or struggle to stay nourished due to intense nausea and vomiting.

Our eating habits during pregnancy are influenced by many factors, and they're also really important. What we eat can impact our baby's growth and risk of birth defects, preterm delivery and illness later in life. Studies have shown that the types of foods we consume during pregnancy can also lead our baby to develop preferences for certain flavours, thereby influencing their eating habits outside the womb. And, of course, what we eat affects how we feel and function, as we experience the demanding task of growing a person or two (or more!), and caring for them after birth.

It's not just about what we eat during or after pregnancy, either, as research suggests our nutritional status (and that of our baby's biological father) leading up to, and at the point of, conception can also influence the health of our child. So how should we go about nourishing ourselves in this season of life?

Giving good and useful nutrition advice is not as simple as providing a list of what to eat and what to avoid. In our present environment, there are indeed particular foods and nutrients that most women will benefit from including in and excluding from their diet in order to support their health and their baby's development.

All of this information I will provide in this chapter, but it won't necessarily help you to nourish yourself. And to hand out a menu of must-eat foods without first addressing this feels disingenuous. You see, so much of what makes a person 'well nourished' relies not on their nutrition knowledge, but their ability to tune in and lovingly care for themselves as they move through life. And too much noise in the world of nutrition, no matter where it comes from, can actually impede our ability to do this.

This is not to say the advice I am going to offer in this chapter isn't valuable – many nutrition-related practices we can incorporate into our routine will be of immense benefit to our body and baby, though we may not have intuitively thought to use them. It's just that, these days, we are inundated with messages from the media, people in our everyday life and health care providers telling us what we should and shouldn't be eating, and what size we should be. An insidious effect of this is that many of us are then unable to pay attention to our body without judgement and simply eat food that makes us feel good, in quantities that make us feel good.

Instead, we have a learned tendency to be self-critical, resist our body's natural shape and unnecessarily restrict our food intake (especially when our body becomes bigger and softer than before, as it does after pregnancy), and this creates a range of metabolic and emotional issues that are detrimental to our wellbeing. In other words, we have a propensity to treat ourselves in a way that actually prevents us from nourishing ourselves properly. Highlighting leafy green vegetables as beneficial won't change that.

And so, before we go any further, I am referring you back to Chapter 1 for a refresher on tuning in. While you're there, near the start of the book, glance over Chapter 2 to remind yourself of the value of self-acceptance and self-compassion. So often in the perinatal period we are faced with developments that challenge our ideals – be it first-trimester sickness and an inability to eat a varied and nutritious diet, or the way our body becomes (and often remains) bigger and wobblier. All the nutrition knowledge in the world cannot compel us to make truly beneficial choices if we are unable to accept our circumstances and act with kindness. If you are already of this mindset, I say hooray! Keep it up.

You may have sensed a shift during pregnancy and found it easier to give yourself the nurturing you require, such as mindfully listening to your body, embracing its changes, eating bountiful and vibrant food, being active in ways that feel good and resting when you need to (perhaps because you know that doing so will benefit your child).

It is not uncommon, however, for the critical and restrictive mindset to creep back in once our baby is born, despite the fact that we continue to require this sort of care. In fact, we may need it even more in the postnatal period, as our body is placed under significant strain while we recover from childbirth, learn how to breastfeed, experience hormonal fluctuations and sleep deprivation, settle in to our new identity, and feel the pull to fit into pre-baby jeans and return to everyday life before we are fully ready.

Admittedly, it's all very well to ask you to nurture yourself attentively and abundantly, but as a new mother it's not always easy to do so, as you will surely find yourself distracted by your baby's needs. That is why this chapter, the one following and the recipes at the end of the book contain practical advice to help you get the nourishment you require with as much ease as possible. First, though, I want you to take a look at your mindset, and if it is not one of acceptance and kindness, try to nudge it that way. In many cases, that is the difference between knowing about the kind of support that may be of benefit during this time (nutritional or otherwise), and wholeheartedly striving to give it to yourself.

Life-giving nutrients and foods

As we grow and care for our babies, certain nourishing practices can help us thrive. It's important to note, however, that all women are different. The way we absorb and metabolise nutrients varies, and we each have our own set of preferences and circumstances that influence our choices. Therefore, in order to get the most out of this chapter (or any recommendations you read), you are going to need to look within and make adjustments to suit your needs. If you are unsure of your needs, I encourage you to seek personalised advice from a dietitian.

OVERARCHING PRINCIPLES FOR PRECONCEPTION, AND PERINATAL NOURISHMENT

- Eat lots of wholefoods.

- Listen to your body.

- Strive for balanced meals.

- Move in ways that feel good.

- Take quality supplements.

- Be kind to yourself.

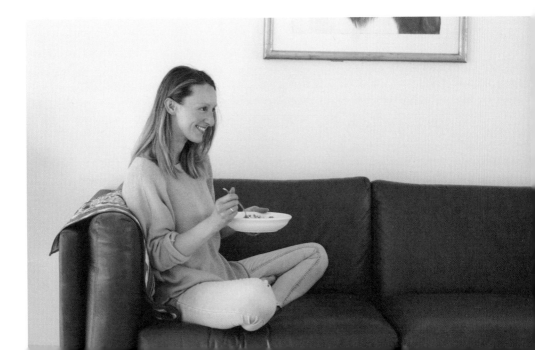

Eat lots of wholefoods

Generally speaking, wholefoods give our body generous doses of the nutrients we need. This is especially important during periods of increased nutrient requirement, such as when growing and breastfeeding a baby.

I define wholefoods as foods that have been grown or raised in our natural environment, and that haven't been processed beyond what is necessary. Now some degree of processing is normal in order to get food from field to plate (cooking is a process, after all). And sometimes additional processing is warranted, such as to extend a product's shelf life. Other times, over-processing is used to cut costs, intensify flavours and sell products; and this can end up altering our expectation as to how food tastes, thereby potentially leading us to consume fewer wholefoods overall. This isn't a moral judgement of highly processed foods or the people who eat them. Food access is an issue of privilege and some people simply don't have a choice. Even if we do have a choice, we shouldn't feel shame for eating these foods. I myself am quite partial to flavoured potato chips. There are, however, so many highly processed foods on the market that our access to them is disproportionate to our access to wholefoods – particularly wholefoods that have been grown or raised locally by farmers who use sustainable practices (yet these are the foods that are important in helping our bodies, and planet, to thrive).

Thus I encourage women to make wholefoods the foundation of their diet (though you probably don't need me to tell you this – chances are that when tuning in you will recognise your body feels better when you eat this way most of the time, and you'll be driven to do so).

Another reason I favour wholefoods is the physiological changes our body experiences in the perinatal period. Many women struggle with a sluggish digestive system during pregnancy due to the action of certain hormones. To help manage this, they will benefit from increasing their intake of fibre-rich foods, such as vegetables, legumes, fruits and wholegrains. Many will also experience nausea and blood sugar fluctuations, both of which can be better managed by intentionally creating balanced, wholefood-based meals and snacks, rather than simply eating a bag of potato chips (which is all I seem to want in early pregnancy).

The same goes for after our baby is born, when breastfeeding hunger and a lack of sleep drive us to want seven cups of coffee and three slices of cake for breakfast. Coffee and cake are excellent additions to our diet, but we won't feel very good if we consistently consume them in the way our sleep-deprived brain instructs us to. All this is to say that you may need to incorporate even more wholefoods into your diet in the perinatal period than you ordinarily would. And that is why I have defined what they are, and lavishly listed a bunch for you to consider on pages 166–83.

Listen to your body

This one is fairly straightforward. It involves paying attention to how you feel and using that information to influence your actions. Say you make the connection that you feel more nauseated when you go for long periods without eating. In that case, you might try to eat more regularly. Or say you recognise you are feeling anxious. Then you can strive to put systems in place to ensure you are engaging in self-care and getting the support you need to manage it.

In the postnatal period, you may notice that you are ravenous and need nourishment, or that your bleeding has increased and you need to see your health care provider, or that you are exhausted and should cancel visitors so you can take a nap. Refer to Chapter 1: Tuning In for more advice on listening to your body.

Strive for balanced meals

When I speak of 'balanced' meals, I am referring to those that contain all three macronutrients: protein, fat and carbohydrate. While it can sound a little nit-picky and scientific, our body works better when the majority of our intake is balanced. This is especially true when our hormones are going wild and we're not getting the sleep we need. When our meals and snacks contain a mix of foods that are rich in protein, fat and high-fibre carbohydrates (as well as vegetables), we tend to have healthier bowels, happier hormones, steadier blood sugar levels and more sustained energy than if we were to eat in a less balanced way (i.e., meals made primarily of just one macronutrient).

Not every meal or snack needs to be perfectly balanced, just like not everything you eat needs to be a wholefood. You also needn't weigh what you're eating to ensure you're meeting specific targets (unless you have gestational diabetes and are struggling to manage your blood sugar levels – then your health care provider may suggest more stringent monitoring). But you will probably find you feel really good when your diet is mostly balanced and wholefood based. Starting on page 166, I have made a note of which wholefoods are rich in protein, fat and high-fibre carbohydrates so that you can create balanced meals without a fuss.

Move in ways that feel good

Physical activity is of great benefit to our overall health. It also helps strengthen the mind–body connection, which is important during childbirth. Find a way to move that you enjoy, which makes you feel energised and is appropriate for whatever stage you're in.

Take quality supplements

Ordinarily, I like to encourage people to get their nutrients from food as opposed to supplements. When we eat, there is a synergistic relationship between the different components within food that affects how each nutrient is absorbed by the body. This interaction cannot be mimicked by creating synthetic versions and putting them in pill or powder form.

While there are supplements on the market that are made using real food, or which contain activated forms of nutrients, we do tend to absorb nutrients better when eaten in their wholefood form. Having said this, there are times when we need a little more support, such as before, during and after pregnancy. In addition, some women are genetically predisposed to require more of certain nutrients, and for them supplementation will be crucial. See pages 186–90 for a list of supplements you might consider taking.

Be kind to yourself

As discussed in Chapter 2, self-acceptance and self-compassion help us to feel content with our circumstances and lead us to engage in behaviours that will benefit our physical and mental health.

Food

Here is a list of foods I suggest including in your diet in the perinatal period. As you read through you will see I have made note of various nutrients. This is not to say the foods listed only contain these highlighted nutrients, or to suggest you need to track the nutritional content of everything you eat. While it's good to be aware of your nutrient intake, particularly in this season of life, it isn't something to become fixated on. We need to be able to eat and enjoy food that brings us pleasure, regardless of its nutritional value (provided it is safe for us and our baby, of course). My hope is that you take this list as inspiration to nourish yourself and your baby abundantly, with a variety of wholefoods.

VEGETABLES

Leafy greens (spinach, silverbeet, rocket), herbs, cabbage, broccoli, cauliflower, carrots, potato, sweet potato, parsnip, turnip, onion, leek, garlic, mushrooms, seaweed, and so on

Try to:

- Eat a variety of vegetables in generous quantities. Doing so will help you reach your nutrient requirements and feed the good bacteria in your gut, which thrive on a diet rich in lots of different veggies.

- Increase your intake of folate-rich leafy greens, such as spinach, silverbeet and rocket – aiming to eat them every day. Folate is important for your baby's development, particularly in the lead-up to, and the early weeks of, conception. Herbs are another good way to get more leafy greens into your diet. You may like to include nutrient-rich nettle in the postnatal period – in tea, soups or stews. Leafy greens are also a source of plant-based iron.

- Include a little onion and garlic in your meals during pregnancy, especially if you want your baby to eat them. Studies show babies who are exposed to these flavours in the womb are more accepting of them later on. The same goes for spices. Pregnancy hormones may mean these foods cause you digestive discomfort, so see how you go.

- Include some seaweed, such as nori, in your diet every so often for an iodine hit. Once a week is a good goal. Vegetarians and vegans may look to an algae supplement to provide them with nutrients pregnancy. Be sure to check with a dietitian or your midwife or obstetrician first. **Note:** It is recommended that pregnant women avoid eating sushi (more on page 209).

FRUIT
Avocados, bananas, apples, pears, citrus fruits, berries, and so on

Try to:

- Keep avocados on hand – they're an easy addition to increase the fat, fibre and folate content of your meals.

- Leave the skin on fruits, where appropriate, for more fibre.

- Keep fruit in your bag for when you need a snack. As your appetite increases, or when dealing with nausea, you may find yourself needing to snack more often. Fruit is an energising and refreshing

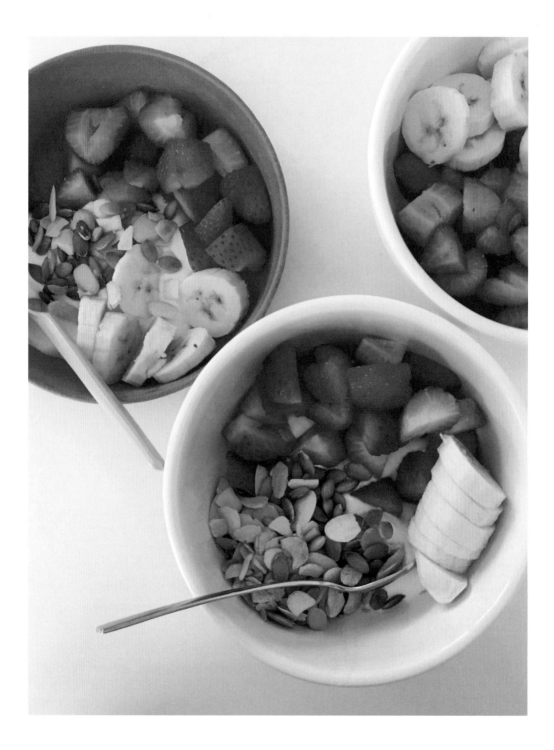

source of high-fibre carbohydrates. Pairing fruit with nuts makes for a more balanced snack, as nuts are rich in fat and also contain protein.

- Freeze fruit, such as bananas and berries, to use in smoothies. Smoothies are a great way to get in lots of nutrients and stay hydrated, and frozen fruit will make them thick and tasty.

- Look for preservative-free dried fruit. Not only do preservative-free fruits, such as apricots and sultanas, taste great, but they won't contain sulphites, which some people are sensitive to.

LEGUMES

Lentils, chickpeas, cannellini beans, kidney beans, black beans, and so on

Try to:

- Eat legumes regularly, if you enjoy them. They are a wonderful source of high-fibre carbohydrates, as well as plant-based protein and iron. Consume a variety of legumes for different nutritional benefits. Vegetarians and vegans in particular may wish to include fermented tempeh (made from soybeans) in their diet as a source of amino acids that aid in the body's production of collagen (more on pages 174–5).

- Add legumes to soups and stews – they're an easy addition and boost the nutritional content. Kidney beans go well with minced beef to make chilli or taco fillings, and you can add lentils to bolognese sauce to stretch the number of servings and help cut down your meat intake.

- Make or buy hummus. Like avocado, it's a great way to bulk out and balance a meal or snack.

- Use legumes as a bread alternative. I love bread, but for variety's sake you might like to make a salad bowl with legumes instead of a salad sandwich. This is a good option if you've already had toast for breakfast and don't feel like more bread come lunchtime. Simply put the ingredients you would have used in your sandwich (vegetables, boiled egg/fish/chicken, pickles, etc.) into a bowl and add some rinsed tinned legumes.

EGGS

Try to:

- Include eggs as a source of protein and fats. Eggs also contain choline, iodine and fat-soluble vitamins A, D and E. For ovo-lacto vegetarians, egg whites are a valuable source of glycine (more on glycine in the meat section on pages 174–5).

- Eat eggs daily during pregnancy – especially if you don't eat meat or fish. In the past, people were encouraged to restrict their egg intake out of fear it would increase their blood cholesterol levels. Studies have recently quashed this concern.

- Cook eggs thoroughly during pregnancy to reduce the risk of bacterial contamination (more on pages 208–9).

- Buy truly free-range eggs whenever possible, to support more humane farming practices.

NUTS AND SEEDS

Almonds, walnuts, tahini, pepitas, sunflower seeds, hemp seeds, chia seeds, quinoa, and so on

Try to:

- Eat nuts and seeds daily. They are an excellent source of fats and fibre, and also contain protein, and many are a plant-based source of glycine.

- Buy nut and seed butters that are made with 100% nuts. These are called 'natural' nut butters.

- Favour walnuts over other nuts (that is, if you enjoy them). They give us more of the great fats we tend to lack in our present-day diet. Look for fresh walnuts that are pale and avoid any that smell rancid or 'off'.

- Store nuts and seeds in the fridge to preserve their life. This is particularly important if buying in bulk, as you may find it takes some time to get through what you have purchased.

- Use tahini in place of peanut butter. I love peanut butter and eat it almost daily, but if you like tahini it's a good idea to include some in your daily diet, too. Tahini is particularly high in calcium, which is great for those who don't consume dairy. If you like bitter flavours you may enjoy unhulled tahini, though the hulled variety (where the outer layer of the seeds has been removed) tends to be favoured by most people. Tahini is incredibly versatile and can be used in making hummus, salad dressings and sauces.

- Include hemp seeds as a great source of plant-based protein and omega fats. These seeds, which you may find in health food shops as 'hemp hearts', are incredibly nutritious and can be added to smoothies, stirred through soup and sprinkled over porridge and salad. Hemp is cultivated from a variety of marijuana plant that contains no, or very low, psychoactive properties. Provided you don't have an allergy to hemp seeds, they are safe to consume during pregnancy and while breastfeeding.

- Incorporate quinoa into your diet. Quinoa is a source of protein and high-fibre carbohydrates, and contains a variety of valuable minerals. Though technically a seed, quinoa is used like a grain – often added to salads or served as an accompaniment to stews. Quinoa flakes can be used in place of oats to make porridge.

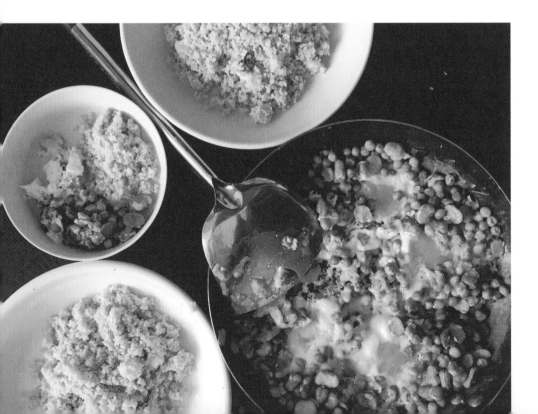

- Toast nuts and seeds in a frying pan for added flavour. You don't need to add oil, simply dry-toast them over medium heat for a couple of minutes until they turn golden, then sprinkle the toasted nuts and seeds over porridge, salads, pilafs and tagine dishes. It's one of my favourite easy tricks to make a dish super tasty.

FISH

Oily fish (such as salmon, sardines and anchovies), white fish (such as flathead and hoki/blue grenadier), shellfish (such as cooked mussels and cooked prawns)

Try to:

- Consume fish 2–3 times a week, as a great source of protein and zinc. Certain varieties of fish will also be rich in fat and iodine.

- Prioritise oily fish for their omega-3 fatty acid content. This is particularly important in the third trimester and postnatally. Sardines are a great choice, as they are also a source of iron and are a more sustainable option. If you do not like oily fish or do not consistently eat them, I suggest talking to your health care provider about taking a DHA supplement (see page 187 for more information).

- Avoid fish that can have high mercury levels. These include large fish such as shark, king mackerel, swordfish and fresh tuna.

- Favour wild-caught fish wherever possible. In Australia, many of the fresh fillets we have access to are farmed, but we do have access to tinned fish that is wild-caught, such as salmon and sardines. The tinned varieties tend to be cheaper, too.

- Eat the bones in tinned fish. They are a great source of calcium and glycine.

- Cook shellfish thoroughly to reduce the risk of contamination by bacteria. Shellfish are full of beneficial iodine, zinc and glycine.

MEAT AND POULTRY

Beef, lamb, pork, turkey, chicken and organ meats

Try to:

- Keep portions modest. You don't need a lot of meat to get a hit of protein, iron, zinc, magnesium, choline and B vitamins – a little goes a long way. It's better both for our bodies and the planet to fill up on plant-based foods.

- Buy grass-fed meat (look for 100% grass-fed, instead of 'grass finished'). These products are not just better for the environment, but animals raised via organic or biodynamic practices can be treated more humanely. It's also a better option nutritionally. When animals are free to roam and consume grass, their bodies will contain higher levels of valuable fats.

- Eat meat cuts that are rich in glycine. Glycine is an amino acid that helps make up the protein collagen. During pregnancy, your body's need for glycine increases to support your baby's growth. Glycine is particularly abundant in the skin, bones, ligaments and connective tissue of meat and fish. To increase your intake of glycine, look for cuts of meat that lend themselves to slow-cooking, such as beef cheek, shanks (such as osso-buco) and chuck. Not only will these cuts contain more glycine than fillet steaks, but they are often cheaper (thus it will be easier to afford grass-fed varieties). You can also use the bones to make stock (see below). Alternatively, you can consume glycine by adding collagen powder to your smoothies, tea, coffee or soups, or making homemade jellies or gummies using gelatin powder.

- Eat organ meats in small quantities. These cuts are highly nutritious and can be a valuable source of nourishment, particularly for women who are low in iron, folate and vitamin B12 and do not eat many other animal products. However, it's important to not eat too much, especially in conjunction with your prenatal vitamin, as doing so may cause you to consume potentially harmful quantities of vitamin A. It may help to limit yourself to a small portion (such as 60 g) once a fortnight. If you are eating organ meats in addition to taking your prenatal vitamin, I recommend checking your overall intake of vitamin A with your obstetrician, doctor or dietitian, as different supplements contain different forms of the nutrient. **Note:** Pâté is a high-risk food for listeria, so it is not recommended during pregnancy (more on pages 208–9).

- Include bones when making stock. Animal bones are full of glycine and, when added to a pot with water and other ingredients (see recipe on page 288), help to create a stock that is rich in collagen. Stock is a wonderfully comforting and supportive food to consume regularly in the perinatal period, while your body is growing and recovering.

GRAINS

Oats, millet, buckwheat, rye, barley, rice, wheat, and so on

Try to:

- Prioritise whole grains (those that haven't had the outer layers of the grain removed during processing), as they will be higher in fibre than heavily processed varieties.

- Consume carbohydrate-rich grains alongside foods that contain protein and fat, for a more balanced intake of nutrients.

- Favour breads that are dense, grainy and brown, like dark rye (if you enjoy them, of course). These varieties produce a gentler blood sugar response, especially when topped with protein and/or fat-rich toppings (such as egg, avocado or nut butter). Sourdough bread is a great option, as it produces a gentle release of energy and is easily digestible, thanks to the fermentation process involved in making the bread. Beware that some breads labelled 'sourdough' aren't made with a sourdough starter and don't receive a long fermentation time (and hence are not true sourdough). Ask your baker about their practices and read the ingredients list on packets.

- Favour basmati rice over short-grain varieties for a gentler blood sugar response. Brown rice will have more fibre than white varieties.

- Eat a variety of grains rather than relying on those you are used to. A varied diet is great for our body. If you're unsure how to prepare new-to-you grains, search online for instructional videos.

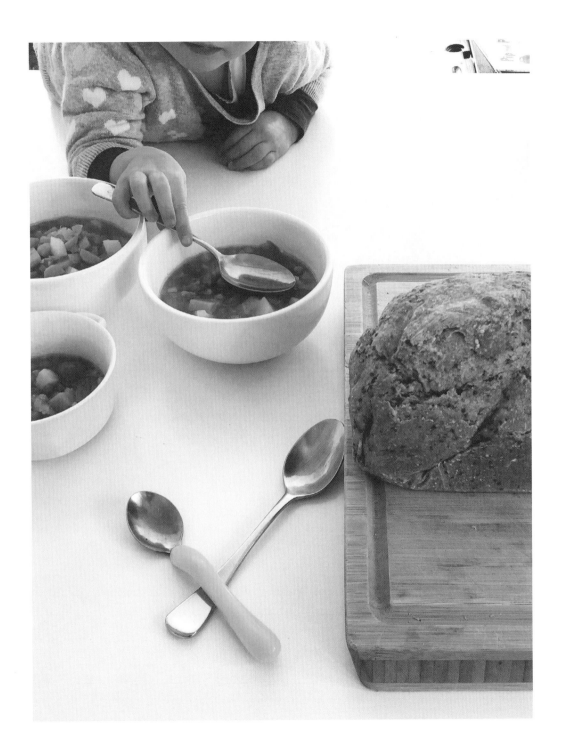

Soaking your grains, legumes, nuts and seeds before cooking and consuming can make them easier to digest and improve your ability to absorb their nutrients. While the practice of soaking may seem like a lot of effort, it is worth considering, particularly if you rely on these foods to help you reach your nutritional needs (as many vegetarians and vegans will), if you have had trouble maintaining good iron or other nutrient levels in the past, or if you are prone to digestive issues. **Note:** Many dried legumes require a soaking period before cooking.

DAIRY

Plain yoghurt, cheese, milk, and so on

Try to:

- Favour full-fat varieties. Studies show that full-fat dairy is more supportive of good fertility than low-fat varieties. Our need for fat increases when breastfeeding, and full-fat dairy can provide you with beneficial fats, along with protein, B vitamins and calcium.

- Favour plain, unsweetened yoghurt that contains live cultures.

- Buy organic dairy whenever you can, for the same reasons highlighted in the meat section above.

- Avoid unpasteurised dairy to reduce your risk of listeriosis. For the same reason, avoid soft cheese or heat it thoroughly until steaming. See pages 208–9 for more information.

- Use real butter or ghee in place of margarine. Vegans may like to use avocado as a spread or even a drizzle of extra-virgin olive oil.

- Cook with ghee. Ghee is made by heating butter and removing the milk solids, leaving only the fat. People who are lactose intolerant, and some who are dairy intolerant, may be able to consume ghee without ill effects. Ghee contains healthy fats and fat-soluble vitamins. It also has a high smoke point, so it's great for cooking.

- Drink a smoothie if you are struggling to eat, whether that's due to pregnancy-related nausea at the start of your pregnancy, reduced stomach space towards the end or an increased need for nutrients postnatally. A smoothie can help you to get a bunch of goodness in easily. You don't need to include dairy to make a smoothie, but it often lends itself to including milk, yoghurt or kefir (see pages 272–3 for smoothie recipes).

A note on calcium: your calcium needs increase during pregnancy, but so too does your body's ability to absorb it. If you consume some dairy products daily, you may find it easier to get enough calcium, but dairy isn't the only way to consume this important mineral. Tinned fish with bones is a great source, and calcium can also be found in tahini, figs, leafy greens and almonds. Try to include these foods in your diet consistently, especially if you don't consume dairy (fortified non-dairy milks are another option). In order to create breastmilk, your body will draw upon your bone stores, which places you at risk of osteoporosis later in life. Thus it's important to keep consuming these foods in addition to dairy (if you wish) and to continue your prenatal supplement postnatally.

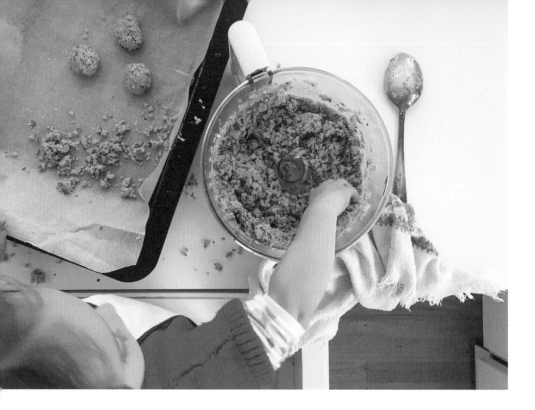

OILS

Try to:

- Favour extra-virgin olive oil as your oil of choice. Extra-virgin olive oil contains high levels of various antioxidants and fats, which are supremely nourishing for our body and may protect us from disease. Good-quality, fresh extra-virgin olive oil is fairly heat stable and can withstand most home cooking processes (such as sautéing and roasting below 190°C). Be sure to select extra-virgin olive oil (not light or other olive oil varieties that have been filtered with other oils), and try to buy Australian, as it will likely be fresher than overseas varieties (the fresher the better – look for a date of harvest on the tin).

- Drizzle extra-virgin oil on your vegetables to help your body absorb the nutrients contained within them. Fat with vegetables is a good thing! It also makes them taste really good.

- Limit your intake of vegetable oils, such as sunflower oil and non-descript, blended 'vegetable oil'. In our current food system, it's easy to consume a lot of these vegetable oils – many processed foods use vegetable oils, as do restaurants, particularly those serving fried food. These oils are often high in omega-6 fats, too much of which (when combined with a low intake of omega-3 fats) may not be supportive of good health. This is not to say we need to avoid all omega-6 fats, as they are found in many nutritious foods. It's simply good to know that we tend to eat a lot of them and could benefit from a) reducing our intake of vegetable oils; and b) consuming more omega-3 fatty acids.

- Avoid trans fats (specifically, man-made partially hydrogenated oils). In recent years, the use of trans fats in commercial food preparation has declined (particularly in Australia), but it's worth checking labels and inquiring as to the kind of oils your favourite bakery or fried food place uses.

- Avoid oils sold in plastic bottles, and don't expose them to heat. Oils go rancid when they come in contact with heat and light, creating free radicals that are damaging to our health. Favour dark glass bottles and store them in a cool place. Some oils, such as flaxseed, should be stored in the fridge.

- Use ghee for cooking. Though solid at room temperature, you can treat it like an oil when cooking (more on ghee in the dairy section, pages 178–9).

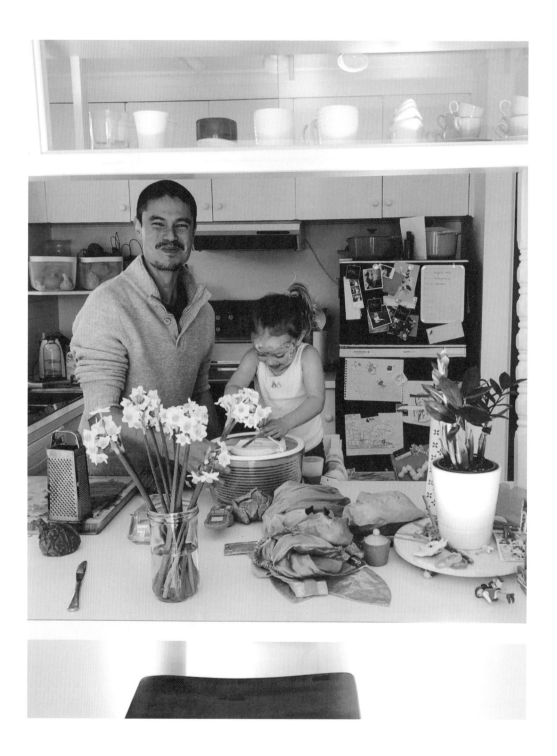

- Use coconut oil if you enjoy it. While this oil has become popular in recent years, I still favour extra-virgin olive oil when to comes to both flavour and health benefits. Coconut oil is a neat product, though, as it's liquid when warmed and solid when cool, and works well in baked goods, date balls and as an ice-cream topping (when combined with cacao powder and maple syrup).

FLUIDS

Your fluid requirements increase during pregnancy, as your body creates, shifts and grows. Getting enough fluids is essential when recovering from childbirth and breastfeeding. A good way to check whether you're getting enough is to observe the colour of your urine. If it's yellow, you should drink more water. Clear or pale-yellow urine is a sign you're well hydrated. As well as water, you may enjoy drinking broth, tea (see notes on page 210), milk and liquid food such as soup.

SALT

Pregnant women used to be encouraged to restrict their salt consumption. Now we know it's important to have an adequate salt intake when growing a baby. Unless you have a specific health condition and your doctor encourages you otherwise, season your food to taste and follow your intuition regarding how much salt to have. If you eat a lot of commercially prepared foods, keep in mind you will be consuming more salt than if your diet is wholefood based.

A note on buying organic and reducing toxin exposure

I encourage you to purchase locally and organically or biodynamically grown food whenever you can. While at first glance it may seem expensive to shop this way, many people find they have access to affordable, tasty, nutrient-rich options when they do a little digging and seek out local farmers and producers. Community Supported Agriculture (CSA) is a great way of purchasing vegetables and meat, as is bulk buying. Every 6 weeks or so, I visit a bulk organic shop, where I stock up on nuts, seeds, grains, legumes and oils, and I try to buy Australian-grown as much as possible! Food access can be tricky for some and there is certainly a level of privilege in being able to shop organically. Some find they are able to reduce their spending by altering their habits. This may mean cutting down their meat and dairy consumption, eating more seasonally and bypassing more processed items for basic ones (reaching for old-fashioned rolled oats instead of boxed cereal, for example). You may also try your hand at growing your own produce. It needn't be an all or nothing thing – I certainly do not eat locally and organically 100% of the time – but an overall shift in the way we purchase can make a difference to our bodies, the local families who grow our food and our planet.

We have become so accustomed to easy access and big quantities that changing the way we shop and eat can seem overwhelming. I encourage you to start small. Focus on vegetables, for example, before moving on to eggs. Ideally, you will make this shift before your baby arrives, as you will have enough on your plate once he or she is here.

It would be neglectful to mention the benefits of organic food and products without touching on avoiding toxins. During pregnancy, we are encouraged to limit our exposure to certain toxic chemicals, such as those found in paints and hair dye. Many women find themselves wanting to go one step further and cut down their exposure to as many toxins as they can. And as long as this doesn't cause you stress, I'm all for it. The Australian government only permits the use of ingredients it deems safe and tries to enforce limits, but we don't necessarily have the long-term studies needed to assess the impact of our ever-increasing exposure to potentially toxic chemicals. Even if you are only exposed to small amounts of toxins here and there, the cumulative effect is worth pondering, especially during pregnancy. Take a look at your soaps, shampoos, deodorant, make-up and cleaning products, and try to choose ones that are free of synthetic fragrances, parabens and phthalates – which appear to alter our body's hormonal balance.

With regard to cookware and food storage, try to favour cast-iron instead of non-stick, and opt for glass containers instead of plastic. At the very least, ensure the plastic you are using is free of BPA and phthalates, and don't allow it to be heated. Reducing your toxin exposure needn't involve lots of money. While glass containers and cast-iron pans may require an upfront investment, they have great longevity. And homemade cleaning products made with baking soda and vinegar are incredibly cheap and effective. Again, you may like to overhaul the products you use before your baby arrives (ideally before you are pregnant) – that way you will have good options to use around the house, and be ready with gentle products for your baby's sensitive skin.

Supplements

Before taking any supplements during pregnancy and when breastfeeding, always check with your midwife, doctor or obstetrician. Our needs are highly individual, and the nutrient content varies from brand to brand. Here is a list of supplements you may consider taking in the lead up to pregnancy and throughout the perinatal period.

QUALITY PRENATAL SUPPLEMENTS

When you can, favour prenatal supplements that contain easily absorbable or active forms of nutrients. They may be more expensive and harder to find than the regular varieties, but keep in mind they'll be giving you more bang for your buck. Look for a supplement that contains biologically active forms of folate, such as folinic acid and 5-methyltetrahydrofolate, as opposed to folic acid. Many people struggle to metabolise folic acid (the synthetic form of folate) and can end up deficient in this vital nutrient. If your supplement contains only folic acid, pay closer attention to your dietary intake of folate-rich foods, such as leafy greens, legumes and eggs. Make sure your prenatal vitamin supplement contains iodine and vitamin D, as studies show many Australians struggle to get enough of these nutrients. If you are deficient, you may need to take an additional vitamin D supplement, depending on how much your prenatal vitamin contains. Talk this over with your doctor.

With vitamin A, certain supplements contain beta-carotene and others contain retinol, the more active form of the vitamin. While it's important to get enough vitamin A during pregnancy, too much is potentially hazardous.

This is important to be aware of if your quality prenatal supplement does, in fact, contain retinol. Dietary sources of retinol include animal foods, such as meat, eggs and dairy. If you find yourself at one extreme or the other – consuming either very few animal products or lots of them, and especially organ meats – check your intake and supplement consumption with your doctor or dietitian. Lastly, check that your supplement contains choline, which is important for your baby's brain development.

DHA (DOCOSAHEXAENOIC ACID)

Your need for omega-3 fatty acids increases during pregnancy. DHA is especially important for your baby's brain development. If you don't eat oily fish (as discussed above), consider taking a supplement, especially during the second half of your pregnancy and postnatally (and especially if you are breastfeeding). If you are a vegetarian or vegan, look for an algae-based DHA supplement rather than relying on plant-based sources of omega-3 fats. Your midwife, doctor or obstetrician may also suggest the following supplements, based on individual need.

MAGNESIUM

Even if your diet contains foods rich in magnesium (such as leafy greens, nuts, seeds and cacao) and you're taking your prenatal vitamin, you may require additional supplementation during pregnancy. Tell your health care provider if you're experiencing leg cramps, headaches, insomnia and nausea, and they may suggest you add another dose of magnesium. They may also recommend you take a magnesium supplement (together with vitamin D and calcium) if you are at risk of high blood pressure and eclampsia.

IRON

Iron requirements increase significantly during pregnancy. Many prenatal supplements contain iron, though additional supplementation is often necessary (especially if you had low stores going into pregnancy). Your health care provider will check your levels as you enter into the third trimester, though if you are feeling lethargic, dizzy and are short of breath, ask them to test you earlier. Some women find they can maintain adequate levels through diet alone.

The highest and most absorbable food sources of iron are red meat, liver and other organ meats (though be sure to limit your consumption of organ meat, as discussed on page 175). You can certainly get iron from plant-based sources (such as legumes and leafy greens), but the body cannot absorb it as efficiently. To increase the absorbability of plant-based iron you can consume iron-rich plant foods alongside vitamin C–rich foods, and avoid consuming calcium-rich foods and tea in the same meal (as these block the absorption of iron). For example, choose spinach with lemon juice instead of spinach with cream.

You may also like to cook your food in a cast-iron pan, as research shows that doing so can increase your food's iron content.

If you do need to take an iron supplement, know that many women find them to be constipating, so you may need to shop around for one that suits your body. Taking an iron supplement every other day, rather than every day, might also help in this regard.

Lastly, a note on helping to increase your baby's iron stores. The World Health Organization recommends that clamping of the umbilical cord be delayed for at least 1 minute after birth (if safe to do so), allowing your baby to receive a blood and nutrient boost from your placenta. In many hospitals and birth centres, delayed cord clamping is standard practice. Nevertheless, it's a good idea to check with your midwife or obstetrician and let them know your wishes.

VITAMIN B12

Vegans, as well as vegetarians who rarely consume animal products, will need to ensure they are consuming a vitamin B12 supplement. While this is always required, it's especially important during pregnancy.

PROBIOTICS AND PREBIOTICS

There has been some interesting research into the benefit of probiotic supplementation during pregnancy. Probiotics can help support a healthy gut, and when our gut is healthy our overall health is improved (including our mood and immune system). When taken in appropriate doses, certain strains of bacteria may bring benefits to you and your baby. For example, some studies suggest supplementing with *Lactobacillus rhamnosus* may reduce the incidence of gestational diabetes. Certain probiotic strains may also bring benefit to your baby by increasing their levels of beneficial bacteria. We need more research in this area before we can make solid recommendations, but after discussion with your health care provider you may wish to incorporate a pregnancy- and breastfeeding-safe probiotic into your routine.

Along with a supplement, you can eat foods that are rich in probiotics, such as kefir, fermented vegetables and some varieties of yoghurt. However, I would be cautious about introducing lots of fermented foods if you weren't in the habit of eating them pre-pregnancy. You may be better off focusing on consuming a varied diet filled with foods that are rich in prebiotics. As discussed on page 33, prebiotics help feed the good bacteria in our gut, allowing them to thrive while also supporting healthy digestion. Just be sure to drink lots of water, as a high intake of these fibre-rich foods coupled with a low fluid intake can exacerbate constipation.

RASPBERRY LEAF TEA

Raspberry leaf tea is commonly recommended to pregnant women as part of their end-of-pregnancy diet, as it may help prepare the uterus for labour. Discuss this with your health care provider and be sure to check the ingredients list to ensure that whatever you are purchasing truly contains raspberry leaves (as opposed to raspberry flavour).

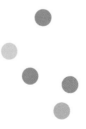

A note on placentophagia

Placentophagia is the practice of consuming your own placenta, the organ produced by your body during pregnancy, which produces hormones and provides your baby with oxygen and nutrients.

Many mammals engage in placentophagia after birth and some people argue humans should do the same. The placenta is rich in nutrients, much like other organ meats; and because it produces hormones, some believe consuming the placenta will help support the mother's hormonal balance after birth. As of yet, we don't have studies to support these claims. In addition, there are various reasons why wild animals would consume their placenta that aren't relevant to present-day humans.

Whether you want to eat your placenta is a personal choice. There is a lot of anecdotal evidence saying that mothers feel better when consuming their placenta, and even if this is a placebo effect, it's a noteworthy one.

If you do choose to eat or encapsulate your placenta, be sure it is handled properly so as to reduce your risk of food-borne illness. Many doulas offer this as part of their service.

Alternatively, you may consider putting the money you would have spent encapsulating your placenta towards a nutritious food delivery service, or paying a doula to support you in the early postnatal period. Good nourishment and rest are vital for the mother's wellbeing, and this we know with certainty.

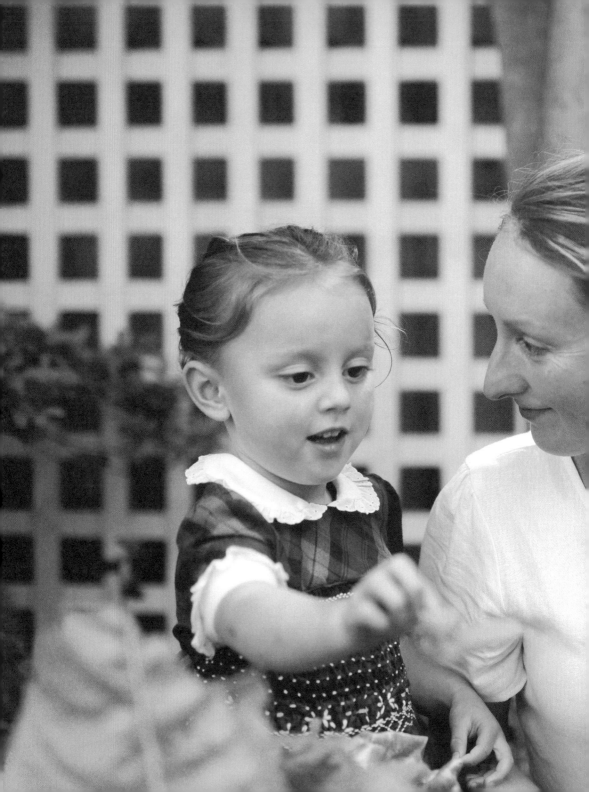

Chapter 7

Nourishing Yourself

PART 2

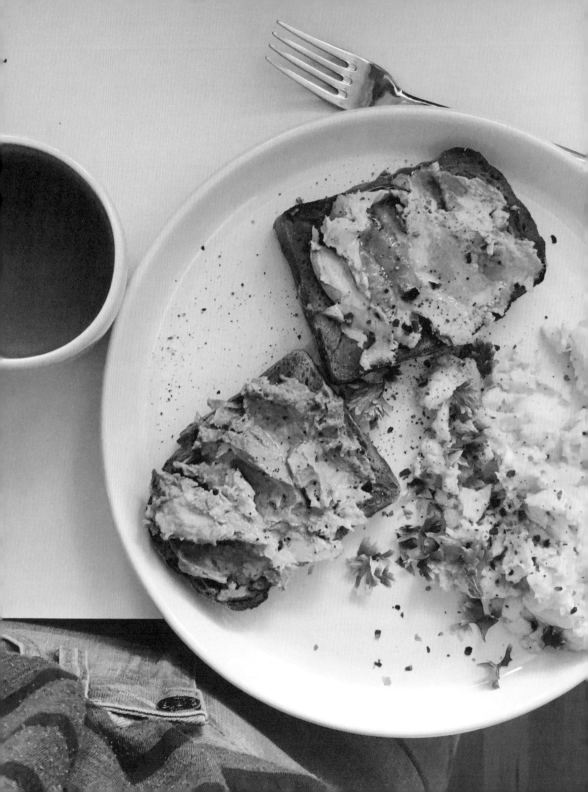

Unless a couple is facing fertility issues, they may not think to do anything special in the lead-up to conception. There are, however, certain diet and lifestyle practices we can engage in to support the process and encourage favourable health outcomes for mother and baby.

Before pregnancy

Studies show fertility can be optimised when we consume adequate fats, protein and micronutrients (i.e., vitamins and minerals); manage our blood sugar levels; and avoid excess stress. Nourishing and caring for yourself in the ways I encourage in the previous chapter (and the ones before it) are supportive of this. Male fertility can also be enhanced through these practices, and possibly others. Indeed, it doesn't all come down to the woman – sperm health is a major factor in the conception of a healthy child. While trying for our second baby, Ben avoided alcohol and ate

75 g of walnuts a day, based on the results of a study I had come across. After we experienced two miscarriages in between our first and second baby, and, with both of us making an effort to enhance our fertility, frankly it was nice to feel as though it all didn't fall on my shoulders.

Research is also suggesting that our baby's health-related destiny is not set in stone – that our nutritional status, food intake, exposure to toxins and experience of chronic stress or trauma during pregnancy can switch different foetal genes on and off, thereby altering our baby's health outcomes. You and your partner may, therefore, wish to make a few adjustments to your diet and lifestyle before trying for a baby. If you're not eating many vegetables, try to increase your intake; and if you recognise your lifestyle is a stressful one, consider where you can make some changes. The perinatal period is immensely challenging, and those with a history of mood disorders are vulnerable to experiencing a recurrence or exacerbation of symptoms. Going into this season, it will serve you to have an established relationship with a counsellor you trust.

Finally, if you simply don't feel well, have a thorough check-up with a qualified health professional. A comprehensive blood test can show you how your body is functioning and whether you need to top up any nutrient stores through more intentional dietary changes and/or supplementation. Having said this, make sure these assessments aren't causing you additional stress. You do not need to eat 'perfectly' or be in perfect health in order to conceive and grow a healthy baby, and stressing about your behaviours will be counterproductive to your goal.

Consider these nutrition-related* blood tests before pregnancy:

- full blood count and a check of your iron stores, and possibly vitamin B12 and folate

- vitamin D level

- thyroid panel.

* You will also be screened for your blood group and antibodies.

Nutrient deficiencies can impact our fertility and risk of miscarriage, so at least 3 months before trying to get pregnant it's a good idea to amp up the nutrient quality of our diet, start taking a prenatal supplement and, if required, have a blood test. If you have been on the oral contraceptive pill before considering pregnancy, it's important to know that it can deplete our body's nutrient stores, including folate and zinc.

Once we do conceive, our body can become further depleted, as it draws upon its stores of omega-3 DHA, iron, zinc, folate, selenium, vitamin B12, vitamin B6 and vitamin A (to name just a few) in order to grow and breastfeed our baby. If we don't watch our intake of these nutrients, we can end up deficient and at risk of experiencing a range of health issues, from mood disorders to osteoporosis. Thus it's wise to ensure your stores are good before becoming pregnant, and to continue consuming adequate quantities via food and supplements in the perinatal period. This is especially necessary if you have a history of low nutrient stores, if you haven't been eating as varied a diet as you'd like in recent months and if you're not feeling as well as you think you should.

You might also like to consider a blood test if you don't eat animal products. Being vegetarian or vegan doesn't mean you are guaranteed to have deficiencies, but some will struggle to maintain their iron, B12 and zinc stores, and may need to check their levels and pay attention to their diet to ensure they are getting enough.

It's not uncommon for Australians to be low in vitamin D regardless of their food preferences and despite our abundance of sunlight, so it's worth making sure your levels are good before conception, as this can affect fertility (this is especially important if you have dark skin and/or poor exposure to sunlight). Vitamin D is also important for bone health, and low levels can increase your risk of pre-eclampsia.

Getting a full thyroid panel done will check how your thyroid hormones are functioning. Poor thyroid function can increase the risk of miscarriage and complications such as pre-eclampsia. It's not uncommon for women to experience thyroid issues in the postnatal period, so this will be one you want to watch.

KNOW YOUR BODY

I don't know about you, but I had a very limited understanding of the female body before deciding to try for a baby. I had been on the pill since I was a teenager, and never paid any attention to my cycle or the fact that I hadn't had a natural one in 10 years. Sex education in school focused on how not to fall pregnant, as opposed to learning about hormones, ovulation and cervical mucus. I had to learn about this myself, through books, online articles and discussions with friends. Looking back, I cannot believe how ignorant I was. And I am not alone – many girls and women don't know the basics about their body's anatomy and how it functions. When trying for a baby, this knowledge is crucial. If you don't know about your fertile window or what is expected of your body when growing, birthing and feeding a baby, I encourage you to educate yourself. This knowledge is important and empowering. The resource listed on page 312 is a good place to start.

During pregnancy

Some women find it easy to nourish themselves during pregnancy, delighting in the opportunity to embrace their burgeoning appetite and fuel their body. Others find it challenging and perhaps even stressful. This section aims to appease some of the concerns pregnant women may have regarding what they should or shouldn't be eating and drinking, and provide tips on managing some of the less delightful symptoms of pregnancy. This advice is not intended as a prescription, but rather to provide knowledge that can be used to inform your personal choices, of which there will be many. Keep tuning in to what feels right to you, and seek personalised advice if required from a dietitian and your health care provider.

PREGNANCY CRAVINGS

I always hoped to experience a food craving while pregnant. Ideally something wacky, like odd foods dipped into jars of mustard or mayonnaise. Alas, that never happened – though certain foods did become super appealing, namely citrus and kiwi fruit.

If a woman does experience a strong craving during pregnancy, it may tell us a number of things. Sometimes nutritional deficiencies or an increased metabolic need for a specific nutrient can be the cause. For example, if our iron stores are low, we may crave red meat. Similarly, we may crave fish for a hit of iodine and pickles for salt.

Our cravings may also arise due to hormonal fluctuations. For example, if we go for too long without eating and our blood sugar levels drop, we tend to crave foods that give us instant energy. Sleep deprivation leaves us more prone to these sort of cravings, too. Eating regularly and consuming balanced meals can help in this regard. You may also want to consider whether you are craving certain foods simply because you have been restricting them, as is encouraged by our diet culture. If this is the case, try giving yourself permission to eat all foods, and trust your body to know what it wants.

Finally, there is a condition called pica, which sees women crave non-food items, such as dirt, chalk, hair or substances that may be potentially toxic. This tends to be an indication of nutritional deficiencies and requires medical attention. If you are experiencing this sort of craving, or are concerned about any cravings you may have, contact your health care provider.

STRATEGIES TO MANAGE NAUSEA AND VOMITING

There are a number of things we can do to try to ease symptoms of pregnancy-related sickness. These strategies may work for you all of the time, some of the time or not at all. Still, they are worth trying.

Eat and drink

As unappealing as food may be when you feel sick, it's important to try to eat and drink. Eating and stabilising your blood sugar levels with small meals and regular snacks can mitigate your experience of nausea.

Try to favour meals and snacks that contain a balance of protein, fats and high-fibre carbohydrates, as doing so will help keep your blood sugar levels happier than if you were to eat primarily carbohydrate-rich foods. This is most definitely easier said than done, because when you're feeling awful the last thing you want to eat is a veggie-packed quinoa salmon salad. Sometimes plain crackers will be all you can tolerate, and that is most definitely better than nothing. Just do whatever you can to incorporate some protein and fats with your carbs. For example, try to have something like egg, avocado or cheese on your toast instead of Vegemite or jam. Eating protein and fats is especially valuable at breakfast, to help you to feel as good as possible throughout the day.

If your nausea is intense in the morning, try to eat something as soon as you wake. Some women like to keep fruit or crackers on their bedside table so they can put something in their stomach before getting out of bed. You may even find an early morning cracker settles your stomach, which will allow you to follow it with something protein rich.

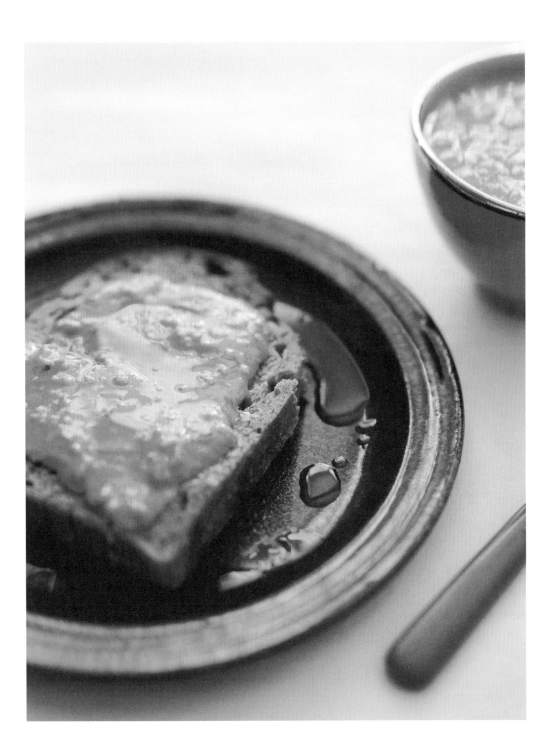

Vitamin B6

Low levels of vitamin B6 have been linked to pregnancy-related nausea. Under the guidance of your health care provider, you might like to try a supplement. Many women find this to be effective.

Ginger

Ginger has long been used to manage nausea. Try using fresh ginger root in your cooking and sipping on ginger water (made by steeping sliced ginger root in hot water). You can also purchase ginger tea bags and ginger lollies. There are ginger tablets you can take, though, as always, I recommend checking the correct dose with your health care provider.

Lemon water and other fluids

It is crucial that you stay hydrated during pregnancy, and if you're losing considerable amounts of fluid through vomiting, ask your doctor or a pharmacist to recommend a pregnancy-safe electrolyte replacement drink. If you're not a fan of ginger, try adding fresh lemon to hot water. During my first pregnancy, I was all about hot ginger water. It didn't do the trick with my second pregnancy, though, but hot lemon water did. If these options don't work, try sparkling water, coconut water or diluted juice.

Ice blocks

Fruit ice blocks can help prevent low blood sugar levels and keep you hydrated. Try making your own by blending fruit with coconut water, yoghurt or milk, and freezing in ice block moulds. Alternatively, look for store-bought ice blocks made with real fruit juice.

Be aware of your nausea triggers

Take note of the things that set off your nausea and vomiting. Perhaps you feel worse in the morning or before meals. This may indicate you're going too long without eating or not consuming enough protein or fat. My nausea was much worse on the days I skimped on protein. You may also be triggered by cooking smells or the sight of certain foods. Knowing when your nausea is worse can help you better manage it. Though it must be said that sometimes there is positively no pattern, it just comes on (or doesn't leave).

Resting and moving

Tiredness can exacerbate your sickness, so be sure to rest when you are able and get to bed early. Also try to incorporate some movement into your routine, as exercise can ease nausea. Even if you don't feel like heading out on a walk, it can end up doing wonders.

Acupuncture

Many women find acupuncture to be helpful in reducing their experience of pregnancy-related sickness. Nausea and vomiting can really take a toll on your body, and it's important to nurture yourself. We also know acupuncture is beneficial in the management of anxiety, which, if untreated, can make us feel nauseous.

Smells

During my first pregnancy, I discovered that certain smells eased my nausea. Diffusing a small amount of peppermint or lavender essential oil worked well for me, as did the smell of lollies. I know it sounds strange, but the smell of lolly snakes got me through many gagging moments during my pregnancies. I made sure to keep a bag of lollies in my kitchen pantry, so I could take a whiff whenever I needed to. I've since passed this tip on to friends and have received feedback that it worked for them, too.

Medications

If your nausea and/or vomiting persists despite trying the strategies above, and if it is impacting your wellbeing and ability to function, please seek assistance from your health care provider. Some like to tough it out, but you need to consider whether doing so is causing you to become depleted or dehydrated. There are medications available that will likely ease your symptoms. This is especially important if you are struggling to keep down any food and fluids, a condition called hyperemesis gravidarum.

HEARTBURN

Heartburn is a common pregnancy complaint, brought on by pregnancy hormones and the presence of your ever-growing baby. It manifests as a burning sensation and discomfort in the chest area, and can occur at any point (though it's more common during the final trimester when your baby is bigger).

Simple ways to manage heartburn, and reduce your risk of experiencing it, are to consume only small portions of food at a time, avoid drinking liquids with meals, and avoid lying down soon after eating. Certain foods might trigger your heartburn (such as caffeine, spicy foods or dairy), although everyone is different and this is not always the case. You may find your symptoms are better managed when your blood sugar levels

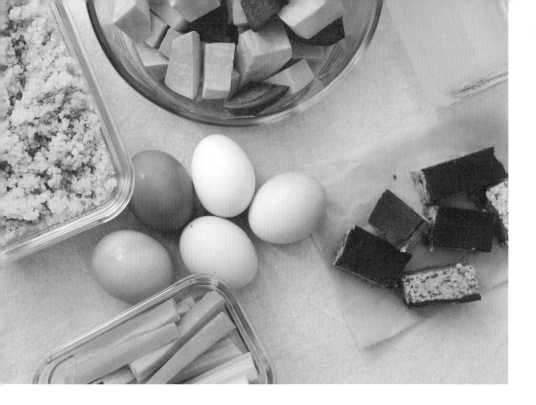

are kept steady, which is yet another reason to favour balanced meals and snacks. If these tricks don't work, consider complementary therapies, such as pregnancy-specific acupuncture. You can also speak to your doctor about taking medication for heartburn relief.

GESTATIONAL DIABETES

Insulin is a hormone that helps to regulate the amount of sugar (glucose) in the blood. High blood sugar levels aren't good for your health or the health of your baby. The changes that occur within your body during pregnancy leave you more prone to insulin resistance, meaning your blood sugar levels may not be as well regulated as usual. If your blood sugar levels are too high, you may be diagnosed with gestational diabetes.

In Australia, pregnant women tend to be screened for gestational diabetes between 26 and 28 weeks via blood tests that aim to assess their body's response to the consumption of a glucose-rich drink. If you have a history of insulin resistance, your health care provider may encourage you to monitor your blood sugar levels earlier than this.

A diagnosis of gestational diabetes requires you to monitor your blood sugar levels at home, and make dietary and lifestyle changes that are supportive of good blood sugar control. These include favouring wholefoods and ensuring your meals are balanced with protein, fat and high-fibre carbohydrates. A gestational-diabetes-friendly diet is, therefore, the same as a regular healthy diet – though women with gestational diabetes will have to be more consistent with their choices and some may find they need to reduce their overall carbohydrate intake in order to have optimal blood glucose control. Good hydration and physical activity are also important in maintaining healthy blood sugar levels. Most women who are diagnosed will see their blood sugar control normalise in the weeks after birth. A diagnosis of gestational diabetes does place you at an increased risk of developing type 2 diabetes later in life, however, so you will need to watch out for symptoms of diabetes, such as excessive thirst and lethargy.

WEIGHT GAIN

Your body experiences many changes during pregnancy. To name a few, your blood volume greatly increases, your body puts down fat stores in anticipation of breastfeeding, your organs move around to make space for your growing uterus and you create an entire new organ – the placenta.

Generally speaking, if you are eating fairly intuitively and being active in ways that feel good, your body will gain the right amount of weight for you and your baby. People in smaller bodies who are lacking in fat stores may find they need to gain more weight than those who have more fat on their body before becoming pregnant. All bodies are different. Some women dealing with first trimester sickness may even lose a little weight initially, and generally speaking this isn't a cause for concern, provided their weight increases later on. If you're unsure whether you're on the right track, or if you're struggling to tune in, respect and trust your body, I encourage you to see a non-diet dietitian for reassurance.

If you have a history of eating disorders and do not wish to be weighed during your pregnancy, let your obstetrician or midwife know ahead of time. Their policy may be that they need to weigh you, but you can ask that they don't tell you the number.

Lastly, inform your obstetrician or midwife if you experience rapid weight loss or gain, water retention or swelling, as this can indicate a medical issue.

LISTERIA AND FOOD-BORNE ILLNESS

Pregnancy suppresses our immune system, leaving us more vulnerable to sickness than we ordinarily would be. Listeriosis is an infection caused by consuming food contaminated with the listeria bacteria. It's rare, but can cause foetal death and is not to be taken lightly.

There are certain ways you can reduce your risk of coming in contact with listeria. These include eating food that has been freshly prepared (wash fruit and vegetables well prior to eating) and avoiding food that has been sitting out for long period, storing food properly, defrosting meat in the fridge instead of on the counter, heating food thoroughly and eating leftovers promptly. Listeria can still grow at refrigerated temperatures, so it's best to freeze leftovers when possible and heat them thoroughly.

You can also reduce your risk by avoiding foods that are more prone to contamination with listeria and other bacteria. These include pre-cut fruit and salad vegetables, sprouts, sliced deli meats, pâté, unpasteurised dairy, soft cheese, uncooked shellfish, food served buffet-style (especially salads and rice that have been sitting out for a long time), soft-serve ice cream, sushi and uncooked egg yolk. Such foods are at higher risk of contamination due to their natural pH level and/or the way they are commonly prepared, handled or stored. I provide this information not to cause you stress or encourage you to restrict your food intake unnecessarily and excessively. A varied diet is incredibly beneficial during pregnancy. Rather, I want to ensure you are aware of the risks and ways you can reduce them, so you can make informed decisions about what you choose to eat.

ALCOHOL

Alcohol can cross the placenta – which means it can reach your baby. Research shows that heavy drinking is related to poor outcomes regarding foetal development, but we don't know the impact of low and infrequent alcohol consumption on babies in utero, as it is unethical to do such studies.

Due to the fact that we cannot claim a safe level of alcohol consumption during pregnancy, the recommendation is to avoid alcohol altogether when pregnant. If you do wish to drink the occasional alcoholic beverage, I encourage you to look into the possible side effects and decide what you are comfortable with. Personally, when pregnant, I would occasionally have a sip of my husband's wine and I was fine with that.

CAFFEINE

Caffeine also crosses the placenta, but at present we have evidence to suggest that only high consumption is linked to adverse outcomes. The recommendation is to limit your intake to 200 mg of caffeine a day, which translates to 1–2 cups of coffee per day. It's important to be aware that the caffeine content of your coffee will vary greatly depending on how it is made. Café-made coffees will often contain higher levels of caffeine than those made at home.

As a coffee lover, I definitely had a cup a day when my nausea wore off. I did, however, cut coffee out when trying for a baby, after multiple miscarriages. Who knows if it made a difference – while the evidence says only heavy consumption can have an impact, some people are sensitive to caffeine's effect on their hormones and will benefit from abstaining. If you drink black or green tea, know that it also contains caffeine, though not nearly as much as coffee. Herbal tea is caffeine-free, but heavy consumption of certain varieties may have adverse effects. Once again, we cannot say for certain, so you may wish to stick to herbal teas that are generally considered safe, such as ginger, rooibos and, towards the end of your pregnancy, raspberry leaf tea (see page 190).

Cacao and cocoa also contain a small amount of caffeine, so keep this in mind when consuming chocolate. Cola-style soft drinks and energy drinks contain caffeine too, sometimes in very high amounts. I don't recommend you regularly consume soft drinks, and energy drinks should be avoided altogether during pregnancy (the same goes for artificial sweeteners).

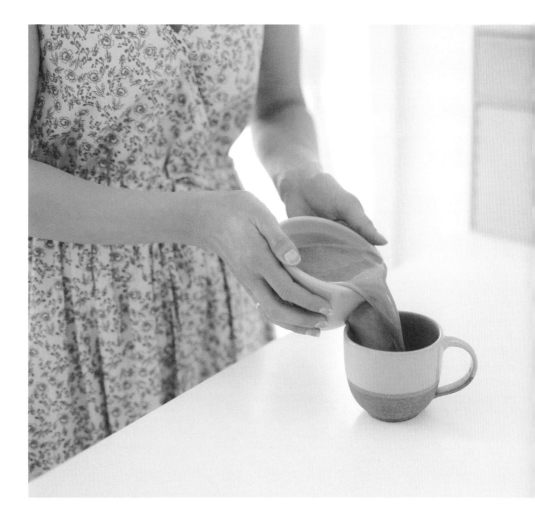

After pregnancy

There are few times in a woman's life when she is in greater need of nurturing and nourishment than after she gives birth. The process of creating and birthing new life is magical, and it is also depleting. Not only are our nutrient stores depleted, many women enter the postnatal period feeling physically drained, particularly if their birth experience was long and arduous. It is crucial, then, that in the weeks following birth, we give our body the chance to recover. Doing so will reduce our risk of experiencing physical and mental health issues that may otherwise manifest and, if untreated, can persist. Replenishing our body with rest and good nutrition will also help us to better manage the everyday strains of caring for our newborn.

When I decided to narrow my dietetic practice to support women in the pre- and postnatal period, I expected most of my clients to be those who were pregnant or actively trying to conceive. As it turns out, the overwhelming majority have been in the postnatal period. This tells me that new mothers aren't receiving the attentive and abundant support they require, and they're feeling the impact.

If you are reading this while pregnant, I implore you to plan ahead and do whatever you can to ensure your future, new-mother self will be well nourished. And to those of you whose babies are already here, know that you need to prioritise your wellbeing. While your little love may remain number one, you need to be right there alongside them.

FOODS AND NUTRIENTS TO INCLUDE IN YOUR DIET FOLLOWING YOUR BABY'S BIRTH

Here is a list of foods and nutrients you may wish to focus on including in your diet in the postnatal period, as your body recovers from pregnancy and birth. Pay attention to these while continuing to consume the wholefoods listed in Chapter 6: Nourishing Yourself, Part 1 (and any other non-wholefood that brings you joy).

Protein-rich foods

Adequate protein intake is important for tissue recovery, wound healing and blood sugar regulation. What this means is that our body will heal better, and we will feel better, if we eat a variety of protein-rich foods in our meals and snacks. Depending on your personal preference, these may include fish, eggs, meat, legumes, poultry, tempeh, nuts, seeds and dairy. Protein-rich foods that contain glycine will help the body to make collagen (a major structural protein). Glycine is particularly abundant in the skin, bones and ligaments of animals, though there are vegetarian sources too (as discussed in Chapter 6).

Vegetables

Consuming a variety of vegetables in the postnatal period will help give your body the vitamins and minerals it needs to recover. Traditional practices favour cooked vegetables for easier digestion. Soups are a great, nourishing food postnatally, as are salads, which can be eaten warm (with roasted vegetables) or cold - however you prefer.

Oily fish

Much of our body's DHA stores are given to our baby during pregnancy and breastfeeding. Regular intake (2–3 times a week) of low-mercury oily fish (such as salmon, sardines and anchovies) and supplementation will help replenish our stores.

Grass-fed, fatty red meats

It's not uncommon for women to have low iron stores after pregnancy and childbirth. While you can obtain iron from a range of plant-based foods, our body absorbs the iron found in meat most efficiently. Meat also gives us a hit of protein and zinc, and grass-fed varieties will be rich in valuable fats (which is why I have indicated grass-fed to be the ideal choice).

Nuts and seeds

Eating a variety of nutrient-rich nuts and seeds every day will help replenish lost stores and give you a dose of healthy fats, including ALA, an omega-3 fatty acid found in plants. It's important to note, though, that the body doesn't convert ALA into the super-valuable DHA very efficiently. Therefore, nuts and seeds are not an equal replacement for oily fish or a supplement when it comes to reaching your omega-3 requirements.

Fluids

Our fluid requirements remain high after pregnancy, especially if you are breastfeeding. Drinking adequate amounts will help you avoid constipation, which will make those first bowel motions easier and reduce your risk of prolapse. Check the colour of your urine to see if you're drinking enough. It should be clear or pale yellow, not dark yellow.

Warming, cooked, wet and gently spiced foods

Ayurvedic and traditional Chinese medicine principles favour these foods over cold preparations, believing they support the mother's recovery and wellbeing following pregnancy and birth. Such foods and fluids include broth, soups, casseroles, porridge, tea and room-temperature smoothies. You may find your body prefers this style of eating and drinking, too. Tune in and do what works for you.

A note on quantity

To help support your recovery, mood and ability to breastfeed, you need to nourish yourself with lots of nutrient-dense food. Some women feel that because their baby is on the outside, they shouldn't have a belly any more, and this can lead them to underfeed themselves in an effort to shed weight. It's normal to still have a belly after birth. Softness is actually good – it represents your body doing what it needs in order to produce breastmilk and nourish your baby. Now is not the time to restrict yourself. In fact, you require as much if not more nourishment as a breastfeeding mother than you did during pregnancy. Even if you're not breastfeeding, you need to ensure you are eating enough to replenish your body.

SUPPLEMENTS TO INCLUDE AFTER BIRTH

Check with your midwife, doctor or obstetrician before taking any supplements, particularly if you are breastfeeding. Those you might need include:

- **your prenatal supplement**: continue taking this for at least 6 months, and longer if you are breastfeeding.

- **DHA**: even if you eat oily fish, I would consider taking a DHA supplement. If you're vegetarian or vegan, go for an algae-based option.

- **vitamin D**: low levels are not uncommon after pregnancy and may increase your risk of mood disorders, so get them checked and supplement as required.

- **probiotic**: this is something to consider, especially if you received antibiotics during labour or surgery. Talk with your doctor or pharmacist about a pregnancy- and breastfeeding-specific option.

- **others as required on an individual basis**: iron, magnesium, etc.

BREASTFEEDING AND POSTNATAL HUNGER

After I gave birth to Joan, I felt the most intense hunger. While holding my newborn, I inhaled a pack of sandwiches, before directing Ben to my bag in search of snacks.

Over the following weeks, I breastfed Joan around the clock and continued to be ravenous and thirsty beyond belief. I would dream of steak sandwiches and chocolate cake at 3 am and devour double portions at mealtimes. This continued for a couple of months before tapering off, though I found I still needed to eat and drink a lot more than usual.

Childbirth requires a lot of energy, as does the production of breastmilk, and your body will very likely communicate this to you by way of hunger and thirst. Sleep deprivation is another reason you may feel an increased desire to eat in the postnatal period. When we experience a disruption to our sleep, our production of hormones is also disrupted, including those responsible for our hunger and fullness signals. As a result, we feel more hungry, more often.

Eating in the way I have encouraged throughout this book – that is, favouring wholefood meals and snacks containing a combination of protein, fat and high-fibre carbohydrates – can help promote satiety and happy hormones. It's also important to eat regularly. When we are over-hungry, any brain fog or extreme emotions we may be experiencing will be exacerbated. Going for too long without eating can also mean you're less likely to get in all the energy and nutrients you need in order to feel well and continue breastfeeding.

If you are breastfeeding, you will probably hear of milk-boosting foods called galactagogues. These foods work to increase prolactin, the hormone that produces breastmilk. In order to encourage a good breastmilk supply, the most beneficial thing you can do is to breastfeed your baby often and ensure you are draining your breast well. Some galactagogues, such as fenugreek, may also help, but if you're looking to boost your supply first check whether you are indeed feeding your baby often enough and that you are consuming enough kilojoules (energy) and fluid.

If you are at all unsure about anything breastfeeding related, contact the Australian Breastfeeding Association (ABA) and consider seeing a lactation consultant. They will be able to put your mind at ease and give you evidence-based advice, including whether or not you should avoid certain foods.

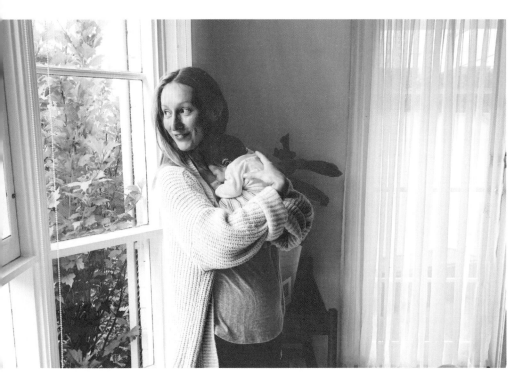

There many old wives' tales surrounding which foods breastfeeding mothers should eat or avoid based on the belief that they may irritate your baby and alter your milk supply. The reality is, however, that there are many reasons as to why your baby may be fussy on any given day, and it is difficult to link this sort of behaviour to your food intake.

If your baby has an intolerance or allergy, this will likely become clear after consistent exposure and negative response (possibly manifesting as skin reactions or a change in bowel movements), and a dietitian will be able to help you figure out what you may need to eliminate from your diet. If this isn't the case, I wouldn't suggest restricting your diet, as doing so can compromise your nutritional intake and cause you stress. It also means you miss out on the chance to expose your baby to a variety of flavours through your breastmilk, which can increase their acceptance of them later on when you're weaning. That said, some women will find that it gives them peace of mind to avoid things they believe may trigger their baby, and this is fine to do, provided they are not being overly restrictive.

Finally, in terms of nutrient intake, it is particularly beneficial for breastfeeding mothers to consume the foods and supplements listed above. Your body will produce nutritious breastmilk regardless of what you eat, but studies do show an increased level of valuable nutrients within the breastmilk of mothers who are well nourished with food and supplements. It's also important to watch your nutrient intake to ensure you don't continue depleting your stores while breastfeeding your baby.

POSTNATAL MOOD DISORDERS

Nourishing yourself after childbirth while also dealing with a mood disorder can be challenging. Often, though not always, depression and anxiety bring about a change in a woman's appetite. She may also feel fatigued or apathetic, and struggle to assemble food to eat. If this becomes your reality, it is vital you seek assistance from loved ones who can help with meal preparation and, when required, remind you to eat. If your appetite is poor, know that it may very well feel as though you are forcing yourself to eat. That's ok – keep going. Good nourishment from food and supplements is an important part of recovery.

High-energy, nutrient-dense preparations for a poor appetite:

- **smoothies**: smoothies are a great way to get in lots of nutrients, and are easier to come at than a full meal. Add nut butters, hemp seeds, oats, spinach, fruit, milk and oils, such as coconut or flaxseed.

- **stews**: stews made with slow-cooking cuts of meat (ideally grass-fed red meat), broth (made with bones, if possible) and vegetables can be terrifically nutrient dense. When possible, add coconut milk for even more energy and fat.

- **nuts/seeds**: keep nuts and seeds by your bed for an any-time snack, and use 100% nut butters on toast or crackers. Nut butter straight from the jar with a spoon also does the trick.

- **avocado**: use avocado abundantly as a spread, in smoothies, in salads – however you wish.

- **oily fish**: fish, especially oily fish, is full of valuable, mood-boosting nutrients. Keep tinned fish on hand for quick meals, like sardines on toast.

PLANNING AND PREPPING FOR GOOD NOURISHMENT

When your baby arrives, chances are you'll be easily distracted, easily ravenous and without the time or capacity to prepare the nutritious meals you so desperately need. Here are some ideas to help ensure you stay nourished.

Batch cook during pregnancy

Spend time in the final weeks before your baby is due preparing and freezing meals for the postnatal period. I recommend making the following: stock made with meat bones (divided into portions so that you have small serves to sip and larger serves for making stews or cooking grains); slow-cooked meat-based casseroles made with the aforementioned stock; sauce for pasta; and gently spiced dhal or other curry. You may also want to bake some snacks, such as mini frittatas, banana bread and muesli bars.

Fill your pantry, fridge and freezer with easy-to-eat foods

Foods such as tinned fish and legumes, nuts and seeds, 100% nut butters, wholegrain crackers, avocados, hummus, cheese, fruit, carrots and frozen peas can easily be combined to make instant, satisfying and nutritionally balanced meals and snacks. Stock your kitchen with these sorts of foods in the final weeks of pregnancy, and keep adding them to your shopping list so you don't run out.

Create a meal roster

If you are having a baby shower, consider taking that opportunity to create a meal roster, where your loved ones can select a date to bring you a meal in the postnatal period. I was encouraged to do this before the birth of my first child by my friend Robin. I didn't end up creating a meal roster, as I thought Ben and I would manage ok. And we did, but my goodness, I wish I had taken her advice. Because even though we had stocked our freezer and our supportive parents were bringing us food, extra meals would have been a blessing.

Back then I felt it would have been asking too much of my friends, but the truth is, they would have been totally happy to whip up a soup or deliver some groceries for us. If you are wiser than I and decide to create a meal roster, I suggest spreading the meals out to ensure there isn't a flurry of food right after the birth. Your partner will hopefully be home in the beginning, and so a meal in week 5 (or whenever they return to work) will be arguably more valuable than one delivered in week 2.

Keep snacks and water by your bed

In the immediate postnatal period, you will probably find yourself living in your bedroom. If you have snacks and fluids right there, you're less likely to forget to feed yourself. Bananas, nuts, dates and muesli bars can sit out unrefrigerated for some time.

Continue batch cooking and meal prepping once your baby is here

After the first few weeks, or whenever you feel up to it, select a time to meal prep and batch cook. This may be once or twice a week, either when your baby naps or when your partner or other loved one is home. The goal with batch cooking and meal prepping is to make it easier for you to consume nutritious, balanced meals when you need them most. Therefore, focus your efforts on meals for the time of day where you find yourself struggling to make balanced and nourishing choices. This may be breakfast, lunch or dinner – or, indeed, all three. Once you've figured out what you want to make, and have all the produce you need, get to it: chop and cook veggies, boil eggs, prepare a batch of bircher muesli or date balls, and make a pot of soup to eat throughout the week.

Plan your postnatal shopping trips

You can't nourish yourself if you don't have food available. Many new mothers fall in love with online grocery shopping in the postnatal period, and understandably so – it's marvellously convenient. If you are leaving the house to purchase food, write a comprehensive shopping list so you don't end up forgetting important items. Many times I found myself wandering the aisles with my newborn, unable to remember what on earth I came to the shops for. If you're still recovering from birth, delegate this job to your partner or other loved one.

Call on your village

Welcome gifts of food and even actively seek them out. Your loved ones want to help, and this is one way they can truly make a difference to your wellbeing. I will be forever grateful for the deliveries of lasagne, soup, quiche, pasta bake and biscuits my family received in the weeks after Joan's and Walt's births.

Pay for nourishment

If you don't have support around you, and if you can afford it, I highly recommend hiring a doula to care for you and prepare you food in the postnatal period. Alternatively, consider paying for a service that delivers home-cooked meals, or good-quality pre-packaged food. Try different services before the baby comes to see what you like, and be sure to read the ingredients lists to see if the meals are a good option. Ideally, they will contain only what you would use when making meals at home. This may seem like a big expense, but consider how much money you might end up spending on takeaway if you don't plan ahead.

Chapter 8
Nourishing Your Family

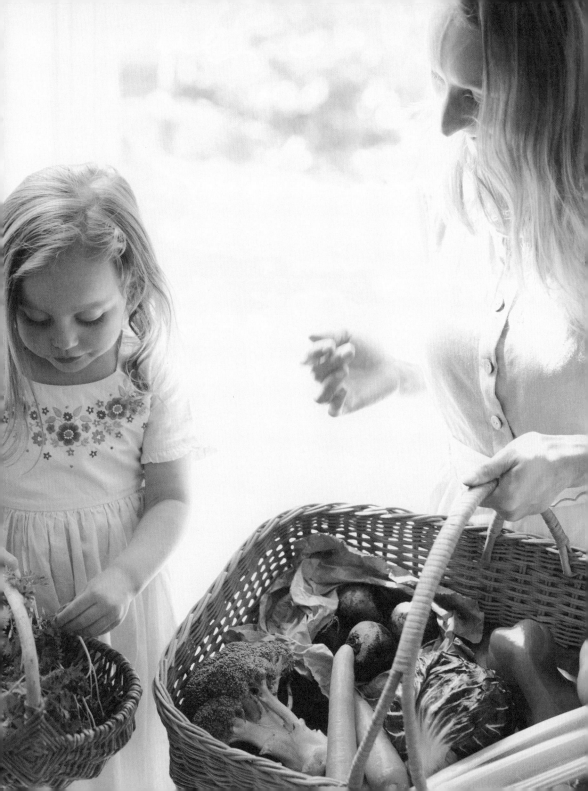

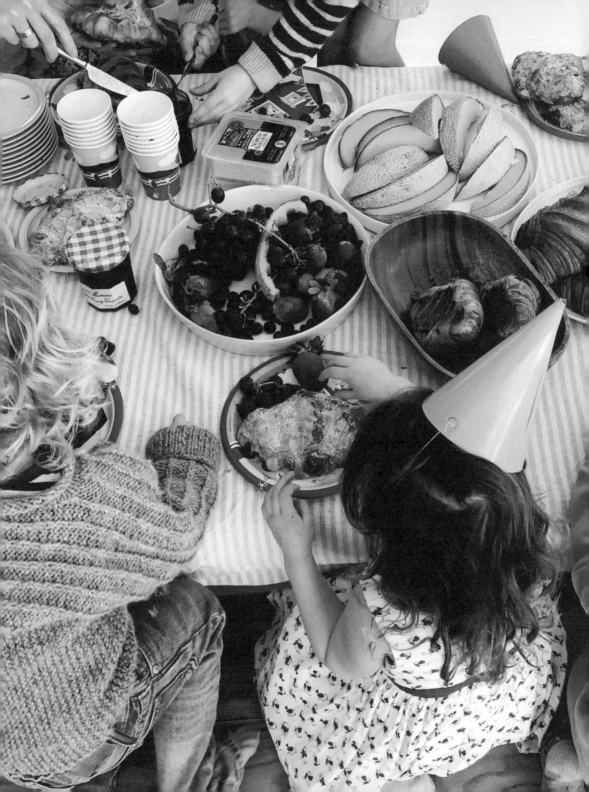

Introducing your child to solid food can be a joyful experience for parents. It can also be a source of tension. Beyond the need to prepare food and clean up mess, parents are faced with the realisation that the way they nourish their baby not only helps their child's body to grow, but can pave the path for their future eating habits. This is an enormous responsibility. We all want to raise children who are well nourished, enjoy a variety of foods and are capable of making balanced choices. That's the goal.

My hope is that this chapter will allow you to feel more confident in your ability to do this, and help make eating an enjoyable experience for you all.

As a dietitian, you might assume I was eager to start this journey, but that wasn't the case. While I love to cook and eat, breastfeeding was, for me, easy and convenient. The thought of bringing yet another task into my days, when having a shower had only recently become a thing that didn't wholly rely on perfect timing, was entirely unappealing. It wasn't until Joan began showing interest in what Ben and I were eating that my desire to see her satisfy her curiosity outweighed my desire to avoid adding something extra to my plate, so to speak.

As it turns out, for me, watching my baby discover the joys of food was one of the most enjoyable aspects of parenting in her first year of life. Joan just loves to eat. To this day, there are few things she enjoys more than sitting at the table with her favourite people and a big plate of food in front of her. Mood permitting, she will try almost everything I offer her and often enjoy it, which makes the experience fun and rewarding.

I put Joan's readiness to eat down to a combination of nature and nurture. She definitely has food-love in her blood, but from the beginning, Ben and I have been strict with regard to how we approached feeding her. We've put a lot of effort into being relaxed about it all, which I realise sounds contradictory, and I'll explain what I mean in this chapter.

If it's not in your child's nature to eat a wide variety of foods, there are things you can do to help them be more adventurous. Conversely, there are also things you can do that may inadvertently lead to them becoming fussier than is developmentally expected. Thankfully, encouraging adventurous eating is easier than it sounds. In fact, most of the time it involves doing less – with conviction, trust and a whole lot of patience.

Let's start at the beginning.

Introducing food to your baby

Babies are first exposed to flavours in the womb through the amniotic fluid. If you eat certain foods often during pregnancy, your baby will become accustomed to them and even show preference for them once they're born. For example, babies of women who ate a lot of garlic during pregnancy have been shown to be more tolerant of this flavour in their mother's breastmilk. What a great opportunity pregnancy is, then, to expose your baby to the foods you hope they will enjoy, and which are beneficial for their health.

After birth, babies are sustained on breastmilk and/or formula until they begin to show readiness for solid food. When exactly this is will be different for every child, though the official recommendation from the World Health Organization is to delay introducing solid foods until the age of 6 months, to ensure your baby's digestive system is developed enough to be able to break down and absorb nutrients. Some parents believe their child is ready to eat at 4 months and will, at this point, begin to offer them texturally appropriate purées. Do not introduce foods before 4 months.

Before you begin, you will need to consider your baby's physical readiness to eat. Signs include being able to sit up unassisted, hold their head up and reach for and grasp food. If you have any concerns about your child's readiness, please see a paediatric dietitian or maternal and child health nurse for personalised advice.

IRON

Iron is an essential mineral that our body needs in order to carry oxygen throughout our body. Babies build up their iron stores in utero and do not tend to need additional iron until the age of 6 months. (See the note on page 189 for how you can give your baby an iron boost by delaying the clamping of their umbilical cord at birth.)

After 6 months, you will want to introduce iron-rich foods to their diet. Iron-fortified rice cereals were previously recommended as a baby's first food, and while these cereals are still available and preferred by some parents, you may consider introducing your baby to foods that are naturally rich in iron, such as red meat, legumes, green vegetables, eggs and smooth, runny nut pastes (thick, clumpy pastes are a choking hazard). As discussed on page 165, there are benefits to consuming nutrients in their wholefood form, as opposed to supplemental (or fortified) form.

For a while it was thought that delaying the introduction of nuts and eggs would prevent babies having allergic reactions, but research now tells us delaying consumption of these foods until after a baby is 12 months old can actually increase their risk of developing an allergy. It is now recommended that you introduce eggs and nuts between the age of 6 months and their first birthday. (Do not give your child whole nuts when they are little, as they are a choking hazard.)

Introduce these foods one at a time, starting with a small portion (¼ teaspoon of smooth, runny nut butter or the equal portion of a hard-boiled egg, for example) and monitor for a reaction. The Australasian

Society of Clinical Immunology and Allergy (ASCIA) recommends you gradually increase this quantity and, provided there is no reaction, continue to offer these foods regularly in your baby's diet, such as twice weekly.

BABY-LED WEANING VS FEEDING PURÉED FOOD

Another practice many are moving away from is feeding babies puréed food via a spoon. An increasing number of parents are choosing, instead, to do baby-led weaning (BLW). The principles of BLW include:

- offering your baby a variety of foods with different textures

- allowing your baby to feed themselves

- trusting your baby's appetite

- sharing family meals

This style of food introduction was pioneered by Gill Rapley, who has written a number of books on the matter. I encourage you to refer to her works (see page 312) for comprehensive guidance about the principles of BLW and how to ensure the foods you're selecting are texturally appropriate.

Importantly, if you are considering going the BLW route, you will need to wait until your baby is 6 months old and developmentally ready to grasp food, feed themselves and handle more solid textures. There are a number of benefits to the BLW approach, the main one being that you can introduce your baby to a range of flavours and textures from the beginning of their eating journey. Research shows this can help them to be more adventurous eaters in the toddler years and beyond. Puréed food is monotonous in texture and, often, flavour. Unless you're preparing your baby's puréed food yourself, chances are they will be consuming a lot of sweet-flavoured purées, as even the more savoury-style puréed products on the market are flavoured with sweet fruits and vegetables in order to make them more palatable to babies. If your baby is used to eating super-smooth, sweet yoghurt, why would they ever accept lumpy, sour-tasting yoghurt? It makes sense to start them early on the things you want them to eat later on, and that help their bodies to thrive – not just the sweet stuff you know they'll like.

Another benefit of BLW is that it can make the parent's life easier. Rather than puréeing foods especially for your baby, you can enjoy a meal together – serving them texturally and nutritionally appropriate foods from your plate (such as the ideas listed on pages 237–9). Sharing food with your baby will remind you to stop and nourish yourself throughout the day (something many mothers forget to do).

The final benefit of BLW I would like to discuss is that it allows babies to have control over their food intake. If we're not physically feeding our baby, and they are permitted to do it themselves, they are free to respect their hunger and fullness signals. Babies and children are naturally intuitive eaters. When offered a range of nutritious foods, they're capable of choosing foods their bodies need and that they enjoy, and eating them in appropriate portions.

It tends to be us parents who get in the way and unintentionally disrupt the process. That said, it's still possible to feed a baby with a spoon and respect their hunger and fullness signals. For example, you can register when they turn their face away from your food offering and stop yourself from coaxing them to have more. It is harder to do, though, as our reflex is to dismiss their cues and get them to eat one more mouthful or finish whatever is in the bowl. If we can sit back and trust them to know what, and how much, of the food we have provided they wish to eat, we can help them to continue eating in a balanced and intuitive way.

I will say that I don't think you need to be a purist about BLW. I understand why people are passionate about following every rule, but I believe that if you follow the general principles (introducing food with a variety of flavours and textures, allowing your baby to feed themselves, trusting your baby while respecting their hunger/fullness signals, and sharing food as a family), then a little spoon-feeding or puréed-food offering here and there is fine.

Some babies may not be interested in feeding themselves at 6 months, and because you need to consider their iron intake, respectfully spoon-feeding them every now and then until they begin to show more interest may be what you need to do in order to help them to get the nourishment they require. Every situation is different, so try to do what feels right for you. And if you feel you need guidance, seek personalised advice from a paediatric dietitian.

A note on gagging and choking

As Gill Rapley explains, the research shows that offering a child more complex textures does not increase their chance of choking – provided they are developmentally ready, allowed to feed themselves and are given texturally appropriate foods. Nevertheless, I recommend all parents and carers do a first-aid course so they know how to handle any emergency situation – whether choking, convulsions or burns.

Before beginning BLW, you will want to familiarise yourself with the difference between gagging and choking. Gagging is a normal part of learning how to eat. When babies take in too much food or begin to swallow before they have properly chewed, they reflexively bring it back up. Watching them do this can be scary, but once they've done it a few times you will see that their body is simply doing what it needs to do. Freaking out may startle them and make matters worse. Instead, remind yourself to pause, breathe and let them take care of it themselves.

If your baby is choking on a piece of food that is obstructing their airway, they will be unable to breathe or make any noise and will require your immediate assistance to remove whatever is stuck. Do not stick your fingers down your baby's throat – this can make the situation worse. Lay them down along your forearm or over your leg with their chest resting along on your thigh. While supporting their head and neck, use the palm of your hand to give the middle of their back (between the shoulder blades) a series of five, firm blows, motioning downwards. If this doesn't work, turn them over and try five chest thrusts (placing two fingers on their chest and pressing down like you would if doing CPR). If this doesn't work, call 000 while continuing to alternate between back blows and chest thrusts.

A first-aid course will instruct you on how to help dislodge the food from your baby's throat properly and allow you to practise on a dummy. This is vital information of which all parents and carers should be aware.

One final note: Always supervise your child when they're eating and ensure they're sitting upright.

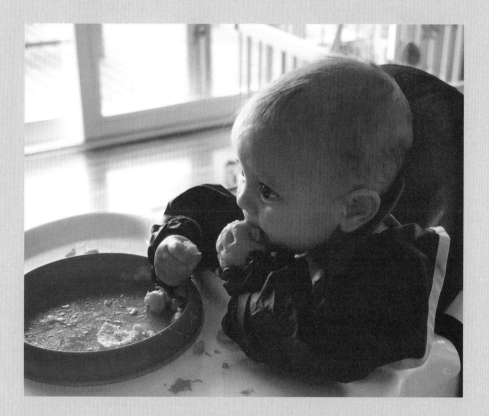

BLW food ideas

To encourage a well-nourished and adventurous eater, try to expose your baby to a variety of nutrient-dense foods that have a range of interesting flavours and textures. Consider nutrition and also consider which foods you hope they might learn to eat and enjoy and offer these. Your baby will take to some foods immediately and other foods not so much, and that's fine. That's normal. Aside from iron-rich foods, you needn't worry about how much they're actually eating in the beginning, as they will continue to gain nourishment from breastmilk or formula.

You may want to introduce foods singly and over a few days, but if you don't have a family history of allergies you could offer them a meal that contains a bunch of new foods. Just know that if your baby appears to have a reaction to something, you will need to backtrack and identify what food may have caused it.

When cooking family meals, select low-sodium varieties of shop-bought products, such as jarred sauces and broth. Once your baby is older, it's fine to season their meals lightly, especially if they don't consume a lot of pre-packaged, high-sodium foods. Initially, however, it's best to add salt to your own meal separately, as their bodies are too young to process it properly. On that note, though, I recommend you make the bulk of your child's diet wholefood based. You don't want to be obsessive about it (you certainly should let them eat cake at birthday parties, for example), but as discussed on page 162, food that hasn't been unnecessarily processed tends to be better for their bodies, not to mention cheaper for you.

For a thorough how-to about BLW, I once again encourage you to refer to Gill Rapley's resources. While sharing a meal sounds simple enough, there are certainly things to consider before passing your baby food from your plate, such as whether there are bones in your fish and if your food contains something they need to avoid, including honey or raw egg.

Finally, be prepared for the fact that BLW can create a lot of mess. Babies like to squish food in between their fingers and slather it all over their face – it's part of the learning process. It helps to be prepared with bibs and smocks, as well as an easy-to-clean mat that goes under the table to catch runaway peas and lumps of quinoa. If your baby is throwing food, know that this is a sign they're not hungry (and/or they've done it in the past and received a reaction, and they want to provoke you again!). Unless you like scrubbing pasta sauce off walls, you're better off saving the meal for when they have an appetite.

FIRST FOOD IDEAS

- **Avocado:** cut avocado into strips or roughly mash it in a bowl and let them at it. A crinkle cutter can help make the pieces more graspable.

- **Vegetable batons:** soft, steamed carrot and sweet potato sticks, or steamed broccoli florets. The vegetables should be soft enough that you can squash them on the roof of your mouth with your tongue.

- **Fruit:** long strips of banana, pear or other soft fruit (i.e., don't offer hard apples). Not all fruit needs to be peeled; in fact, leaving a little peel or skin on the fruit can help your baby grip the fruit and self-feed.

- **Meat:** red meat is an excellent source of highly absorbable iron, among other nutrients such as zinc and vitamin B12. This is particularly valuable for babies who self-feed, as they tend to eat smaller volumes than those who are spoon-fed and, as a result, research shows they may not get enough of these important nutrients. Soft meats, such as slow-cooked beef or lamb tend to be easy to consume, and when these are served in a casserole-style meal your child can consume the nutritious cooking juices. Alternatively, your baby may enjoy sucking on a strip of tender steak or a lamb chop 'lollipop'. If serving your baby poultry, go for the darker pieces, such as the thigh, as they contain more iron than the breast.

- **Fish:** low-mercury fish that has been cooked and flaked into pieces, or formed into patties. Oily fish, such as salmon and sardines, are high in omega-3 fats, which are crucial for brain development. Always check for bones before you serve fish to your baby.

- **Egg:** scrambled, fried, boiled, poached or an omelette cut into strips. Cook eggs thoroughly when your baby is young to reduce the risk of bacterial contamination.

- **Meals:** casseroles with slow-cooked meat, thick soups, bolognese, gently spiced dhal, omelettes, frittatas, smoothies, hummus with steamed vegetable sticks for dipping.

- **Natural yoghurt:** choose varieties without any added sugar.

- **Pikelets or baked fritters:** mini pancakes or fritters made with fruit, vegetables and whisked egg (plus a little flour, perhaps, depending on the recipe) make excellent finger food.

- **Porridge:** soak your baby's oats in water overnight in the fridge, as this can help with their digestion and nutrient absorption. Cook on the stove using water, then cool before serving. Provided it's tolerated, you may choose to cook your baby's porridge with milk (such as organic cow's milk or unsweetened non-dairy milk) or stick with water. You can even bake porridge into strips for babies to grab and gnaw on.

WHAT WE DID

Ben and I offered Joan her first taste of solid food at 6 months, starting with avocado. Initially she was disinterested – casting it aside after a quick lick. The following day she had a little nibble but preferred rubbing it on her face. A couple of days later I gave her some steamed broccoli florets, which she seemed to enjoy more than the avocado. Next up was steamed carrot followed by banana. Joan gagged on both the broccoli and the carrot. Having completed a first-aid course, I knew she wasn't choking. I also knew that gagging was a normal part of learning how to eat. Nevertheless, it was scary to watch. As she learned to eat, Joan gagged less and less, and I found it less unsettling when she did, seeing how capable she was of handling it herself.

This vegetable and fruit introduction took about a week or so, after which we moved on to beef for a bigger hit of iron. Our favourite method was slow-cooking (see the recipe on pages 296–7), as this ensured the meat was soft and easy to manage. Slow-cooked casseroles also froze well, which meant I could always have a nutrient-dense meal on hand. Once we'd introduced Joan to beef casseroles, we began offering her food from our plate that was texturally appropriate. Oats at breakfast, avocado at lunch, fish and vegetables at dinner, and so on. For the first month or so she didn't eat three meals a day; that is something we built up to gradually. We made sure Joan had a taste of nut butter and egg (as outlined on page 230), and eventually incorporated my father's homemade sourdough bread. I didn't worry too much about bread or other stodgy foods like potato and pasta, though. I felt these were foods she would probably learn to love easily, as they're fairly bland and readily accepted by kids, and I wanted her to get used to more complex flavours first. Vegetables, eggs, meat and legumes are also, generally speaking, richer in nutrients, which is an important consideration when little tummies aren't eating very much. They also encourage good gut health, which is crucial in the first few years of a child's life.

The final two foods I made sure to incorporate fairly early on were quinoa and legumes – the latter in the form of plain black beans, hummus and gently spiced lentils. These were a priority for me because they're foods I eat often, and I wanted to be able to share them with Joan. They also contain iron and zinc, which I felt would be useful in helping her reach her nutritional requirements. When cooking quinoa (and other grains), I try to use homemade chicken stock (see the recipe on pages 288–9), as this amps up the flavour and nutritional value.

In terms of portions, I would serve up a few strips or a couple of tablespoons worth of food, then follow Joan's lead. If she was still hungry or really enjoyed something, she would ask for more and I would give it to her.

Only a couple of times did she refuse to eat entirely. Interestingly, this happened when I had served a food I knew she enjoyed and could tolerate – so I took it to mean she simply wasn't hungry. When I served the food again in an hour or so, she had more of an appetite and ate it.

Ben and I strive to have family meals as often as possible. When Joan was first learning how to eat, sitting together at the table allowed her to observe our eating behaviour and copy us. Sometimes, we found ourselves exaggerating our chewing motions and noises, which was perhaps unnecessary, but she seemed to enjoy the show. There are many benefits to family meals, which I will discuss on page 254–5.

Joan made my job easy. She found eating fun and would devour most of what I served her (though her favourites were undoubtedly broccoli, slow-cooked beef cheeks and banana pancakes). Even so, when she was trying new foods for the first, second or third time, she would often put it to her mouth and shake her head as if to say, 'Nooooooo!' With time, however, she would come around. Some things, like blueberries, took just a couple of months. Other things, like leafy greens, capsicum and cheese, took years.

Joan is a toddler now, and while she has certainly presented us with normal, challenging behaviours, she continues to respond to the methods Ben and I use to foster adventurous and balanced eating habits. What are these methods? I'll tell you now.

Encouraging babies and toddlers to eat well

DIVISION OF RESPONSIBILITY, EXPOSURE AND MODELLING

When it comes to raising healthy eaters, parents need to know, and feel confident in, their role, and understand the role of their child. Dietitian and family therapist Ellyn Satter has made things clear for us with her term Division of Responsibility (sDOR), which is now the gold standard on the matter. The sDOR states that your responsibility as a parent is to decide what food to provide your child, when to provide it and where; it is your child's responsibility to decide whether to eat the food and how much.

What I love about the sDOR is that it allows children to go at their own pace. You see, most children take time to accept certain foods and flavours, and as parents we tend to see this as an indication that we need to take action. Yet from an evolutionary standpoint, a little apprehension makes sense. Not all foods were safe to eat back in the day. Bitter flavours often meant a food was poisonous, and this cautious instinct persists today. It's helpful, then, to expect your child to be wary of unfamiliar flavours, and not let this deter you or lead you to think your child is fussy.

Resist the urge to label them a 'fussy eater' and only serve food they immediately like. Remember, part of your role as a parent is to decide what to serve your child, and the more they see a certain food, the more they see you enjoying it, and the less pressure they feel to eat it themselves, the more likely they are to try it. This is called 'exposure' and 'modelling'.

The fact that kids learn to love foods that aren't naturally appealing to their tastebuds (such as pungent, fermented pastes) shows us the influence repeated exposure and modelling can have over a child's food preferences. If your child doesn't touch what's on their plate, reassure yourself that you're not wasting your time. It can take 10, 20, even 50 exposures before they accept something new, and even then they may not eat it consistently. So keep serving it up. And get really good at repurposing leftovers – package them up for you or your partner to eat the following day, or present them to your child at a different meal with the goal of repeated exposure.

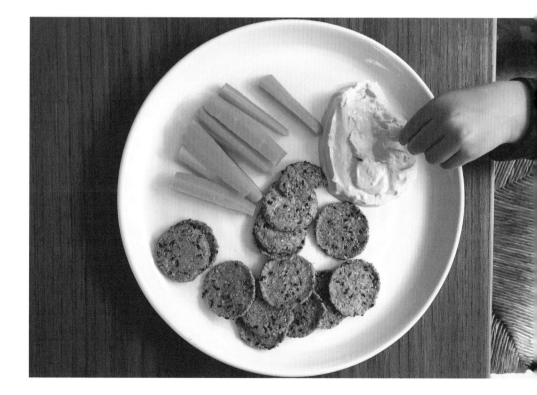

Parents also need to know that it's normal for children to reject food for reasons other than wariness. Many toddlers go through a developmental stage that sees them striving to exert control over their life, and this can manifest in a refusal to eat. Unfortunately, this stage can coincide with the age when they become more reliant on food for their nutritional intake (as opposed to breastmilk or formula), which is why some parents begin to stress about their child's eating habits and throw the sDOR out the window. The best thing you can do in this situation is not show your concern. As tempting as it can be to encourage, beg or bribe, or to make them a meal you know they will accept, calmly continue with the sDOR – that is, you decide what food is served, when and where, and you allow them to decide whether to eat and how much. If they are hungry and sense no pressure from you to eat (if they believe you don't mind whether they do or don't), they are more likely to fill their belly.

Some parents find a 'one-bite' policy works to encourage their child to try new food, but this can also cause children to rebel, especially those in the 1–4 years age bracket. Even my 'easy eater' daughter will refuse to taste a new food if I ask her to do so, but if I let her discover it on her own, she will invariably have a lick, and may end up eating part or all of it. If your child gets upset by the sight of a food on their plate they don't recognise or like, reassure them that they don't have to eat it just because it's on their plate. Know your role and make sure they know theirs.

If you find yourself tempted to coerce your child to eat, know that while it may get you short-term wins, it is counterproductive to the larger goal of raising a healthy eater. When we teach a child to clean their plate without considering their appetite (say, if they learn to eat for praise or to get dessert), we teach them to disregard how food makes them feel. In order to eat in a balanced way, children need to be in touch with their hunger and fullness signals. We can help them retain their ability to eat intuitively by practising the sDOR and allowing them to learn how to regulate their intake. This relates to all foods, whether vegetables or lollies.

Parents are often unsure how to handle food that is commonly labelled 'junk', and the truth is, the way you approach these sort of foods can influence your child's ability to self-regulate their intake. The first step is not to call it 'junk'. In fact, remove all moral labels from food – that means stop saying something is 'good' or 'bad'. This allows children simply to focus on how food feels in their body.

I am not suggesting you regularly open bags of lollies and let them go wild – after all, most kids love lollies and many will eat lots of them every day if given the chance – but you can use the opportunity when lollies are around to make the experience an enjoyable one, without inciting a 'scarcity mindset'. By that I mean, if you overly restrict their intake of these foods or only provide them as rewards for desirable behaviour, your child will learn that these irresistibly delicious foods are so rarely available that they had better overeat them when they get the chance.

If, on the other hand, you provide these foods occasionally, don't make a big deal out if it, and model eating the food in wise portions; they will learn to do the same. Trust your child. Sure, they may sometimes get excited, eat too much and get a bellyache, but don't we all? And these are actually important lessons that teach them what happens when they don't listen to their body. I, for one, will never forget the time I learned what happens when you eat too many dried apricots. Soon after Joan turned 3 she discovered lollipops and promptly fell in love. Every day, upon waking, she would ask for one. Rather than tell her that they were a 'sometimes food', I tried to not make a big deal out of it. I bought a bag (opting for a brand that didn't use artificial colours or flavours) and incorporated them into her snack plates every now and then (pairing them with fat and protein-rich foods such as nut butter, boiled eggs and chickpeas, to help stunt the blood sugar spike). Initially, she would go straight for the lollipop and lick the stick clean before moving on to the other foods. After a while, though, she became less interested. Occasionally, she would even leave the lollipop half-eaten. And that's because she was listening to her body. She was eating intuitively.

Another reason we shouldn't pressure our children to eat is that when we force them to finish a food they dislike, it sets them up to despise that food later in life. What's more, these battles tend to revolve around a food we really want kids to learn to love. Indeed, a surefire way to raise a broccoli-hater is to force them to eat it as a child.

Some babies will move from having breastmilk or formula to eating spiced vegetable stews with anchovies and a side of greens without a fuss. The majority won't, however. Certainly not immediately. But that's ok. That's actually liberating! Knowing that wariness and refusal is normal makes it easier for us to take the pressure off our children to eat 'perfectly', and off ourselves to ensure they do.

Nutrition is important, of course. But in order to raise a healthy eater we need to focus not just on what our child is eating today, but on the endgame – and consider how our language and behaviour can help or hinder this.

WAYS TO ENCOURAGE YOUR CHILD TO EAT THE FOOD YOU SERVE

Come to meals with an appetite

Ensure your child is hungry before they sit down to eat. If they haven't filled up on snacks, they are more likely to eat what you have served. I find that when Joan doesn't have an appetite, she will focus on just one food (whatever she has decided is her favourite that day) and leave, or play with, the rest.

I appreciate that this suggestion can sometimes backfire, such as when meals take longer to prepare than predicted and children cross over from hungry to hangry. If I sense this may happen, I offer vegetable sticks to munch on. If Joan is really hungry, she'll eat them.

Involve them in the process

Kids are more likely to eat a meal if they feel some ownership over it. This may mean you decide on a recipe together, take them to the shops to buy food, pick vegetables from the garden, have them help with the preparation or cooking of the meal, or even just let them set the table.

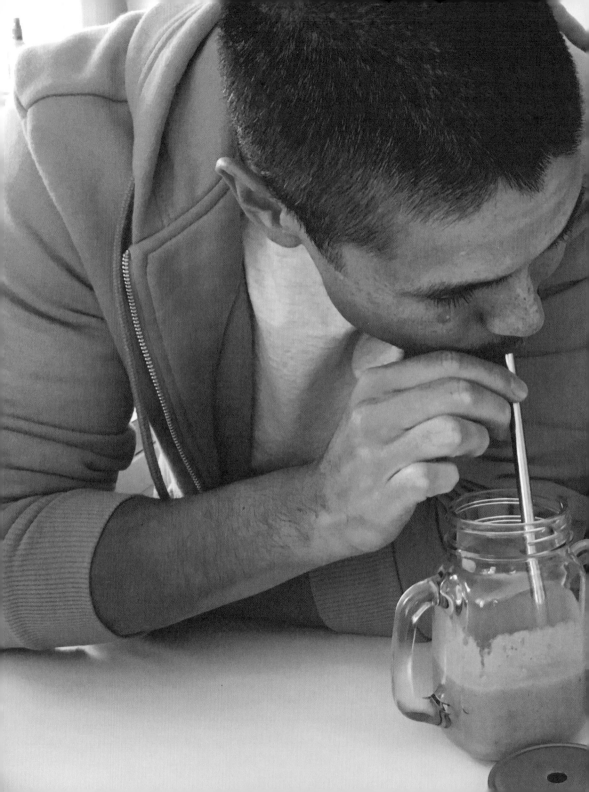

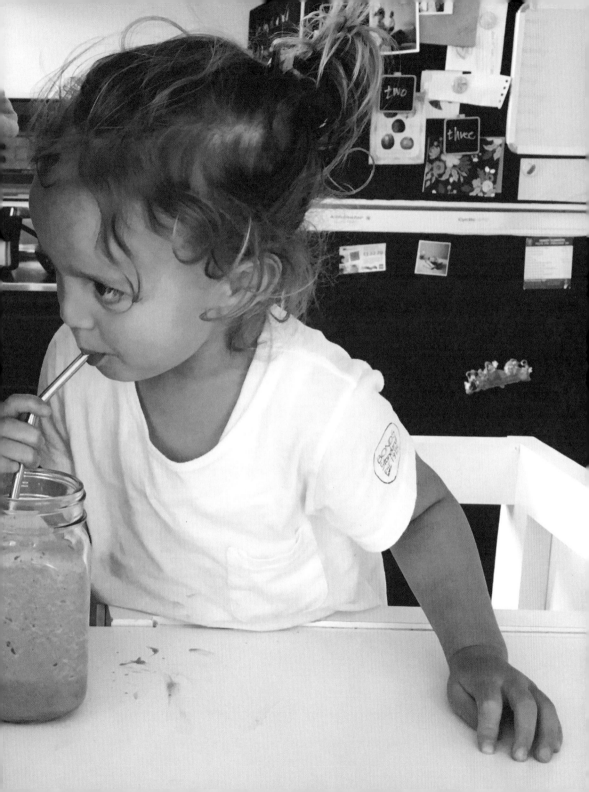

Make it delicious

This may sound like an obvious thing to say, but we can often find ourselves in a rut, cooking the same old method and perhaps even skimping on tasty fats like butter and oil due to the influence of our diet culture. This is such a shame because fat equals flavour, and can actually help us to better absorb some of the nutrients within certain foods, such as vegetables. Try serving vegetable sticks with dip, roasting vegetables with olive oil, making vegetable stirfries with yummy sauces and topping steamed vegetables with butter.

Provide structure and predictability

Some kids are more likely to eat a meal if they know what's coming. You may like to tell them the menu ahead of time or even stick to a weekly schedule, such as meat-free Mondays and taco Tuesdays.

Serve the meal family style

Kids love to serve themselves. Once again it gives them ownership over their choices and satisfies their desire for control. When they're old enough, try placing the various components of your meal in serving dishes – the casserole in one, couscous in another, plus a salad with the dressing on the side in a jug from which they can easily pour – then place it all on the table and allow them to spoon what they like onto their plate. Just remember that it's ok if they don't sample everything initially and instead fill up on one food. Which takes me to my next point ...

Always make sure you have something on the table you know your child likes

This is really important, especially when you're introducing something new. Meltdowns can easily happen when all the food on a child's plate is unfamiliar (I learned this the hard way). If you can present a very small portion of new food alongside your child's favourites (and, importantly, don't pressure them to eat it), there's a better chance they'll come around to it.

Don't make them something else

An important rule in our house is 'this is dinner'. What this means is that if Joan doesn't like what I have provided, she doesn't get an alternative. As per the point above, I always make sure there is something on the table I know she likes and will always eat (sweet potato, pasta or black beans, for example) and if she doesn't want the other components of the meal, that's fine, she doesn't have to eat them. But she won't be getting anything else. This may sound a little harsh, but one meal every now and then where she eats nothing but plain pasta won't hurt her.

If kids know they can get an alternative, they will play that card as often as they can. Not only does this create more work for you, it gives them no incentive to try what's in front of them. If you calmly and compassionately tell them that you hear what they're saying, but that 'this is dinner', they will get the message.

Model eating the food yourself

This is such an important step and far more powerful than talking about why we might want to eat certain foods (which is not always appropriate when children are little). If a child sees you nourishing yourself by munching on carrot sticks, dipping crackers into hummus and enjoying a bowl of soup, they will internalise that image and strive towards similar behaviour.

SNEAKING VEGETABLES

Some people believe sneaking vegetables into their child's food is a great thing to do, and will happily add grated vegetables to bolognese, spinach to smoothies and beetroot to chocolate cake. Others are less keen on this practice, as it doesn't teach children to eat the food they're so keenly attempting to sneak in. Personally, I like to do both – I certainly do a lot of exposing, and I also occasionally sneak things in. I feel that in meals where it works, hiding vegetables can be a great way of increasing the nutrient content of your child's diet. It's paramount, however, that you continue presenting the actual food to your child so they get the benefit of repeated exposure (i.e., if you hide zucchini in your pasta sauce, be sure to also serve your child a side of undisguised zucchini).

You may find that by knowing you've successfully snuck a few extra veggies into your child's favourite meal, you're able to feel more relaxed at mealtimes when they leave the vegetable portion untouched and give them the time they need to develop a taste for it. If this is the case, I say go for it.

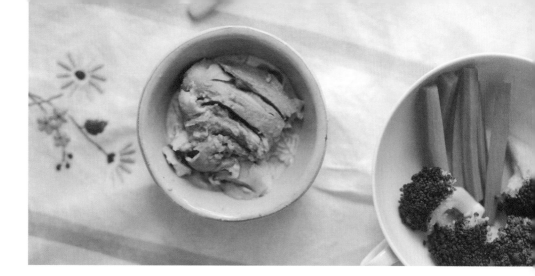

A FINAL NOTE

All children are different. Some respond easily to exposure and modelling; others are more stubborn, have firm preferences and take many more exposures before they'll even consider looking at certain foods. There are also some children who have sensory issues and are more sensitive than the average child to certain flavours, smells and textures. For these children, and their parents, food introduction can be really tricky.

You know your child best. If you have adopted the sDOR, are practising exposure and modelling, have given it lots of time and feel it isn't working, I encourage you to seek the help of a paediatric dietitian. Stressful mealtimes are hard, and if you can feel confident about how to approach the food thing, the entire experience will be far more pleasant and productive for everyone. That way, even if your child doesn't turn into a spinach lover, you can still strive to enjoy the multitude of benefits that family mealtime brings.

Family meals

There's an old Italian saying – *A tavola non si invecchia* – which roughly translates to, 'At the table, one does not grow old.' What this proverb is talking about is the magical power of sharing meals with loved ones and the positive influence it can have on our wellbeing.

I don't want to romanticise the notion of family meals, because the truth is, feeding your family doesn't always feel magical. When you're rushing to put a meal on the table following after-school activities and hangry kids are whining at your side, it can feel like a chore – especially when they complain and only eat a portion of what you prepared.

Nevertheless, the act of sitting at the table and eating a meal together is powerful, helping to foster lifelong healthy habits and connection as a family. Kids crave consistency. After spending their days growing, learning and adventuring, the ritual of coming together to eat as a family offers predictability and comfort. Far more than just an opportunity to eat, these mealtimes allow children the chance to discuss things that are on their mind. It also encourages the development of empathy, as they listen to other family members talk about their experiences.

Whether you sit together for breakfast, lunch or dinner, research confirms that regular family mealtimes are important for kids of all ages. Young children are more likely to eat a wide variety of nutritious foods if they observe family members doing the same; and older kids who eat meals with their family are less likely to engage in 'high-risk behaviours' (such as drugs, alcohol, violence and extreme weight-control measures) and more likely to do well at school. And it's not just children who benefit from family meals – people of all ages thrive when they feel part of a unit. As you can see, you don't just nourish your family by serving them food. Nourishment also comes from consistency and connection – from gathering, sitting together and letting each other know that you are all seen and important and loved.

I will note, though, that I wouldn't expect young children to sit through an entire meal. Most toddlers are itching to get up and run around not too long after sitting down. While I'm all for encouraging good table manners, I would simply let little ones know that if they get up, that means they are finished and their food will be put away. If they're ok with that, and they're truly done, then that's fine. When they're older, they can wait until everyone has finished eating before asking to leave the table.

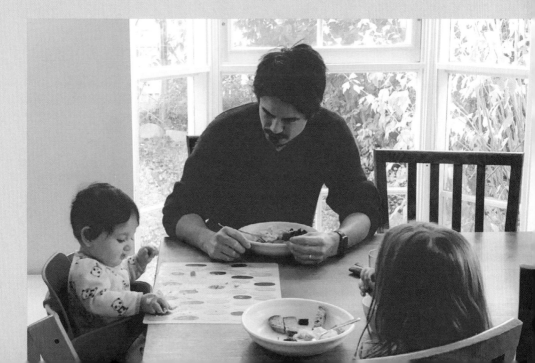

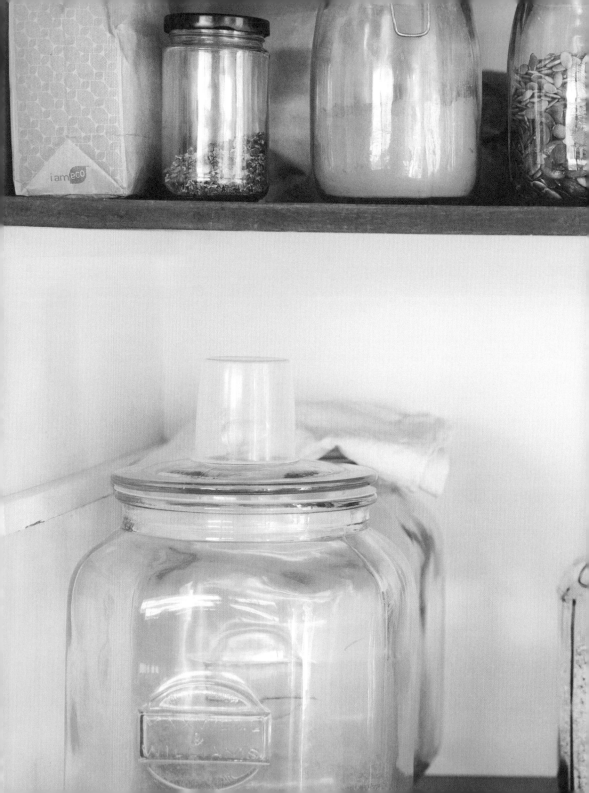

Chapter 9
Recipes

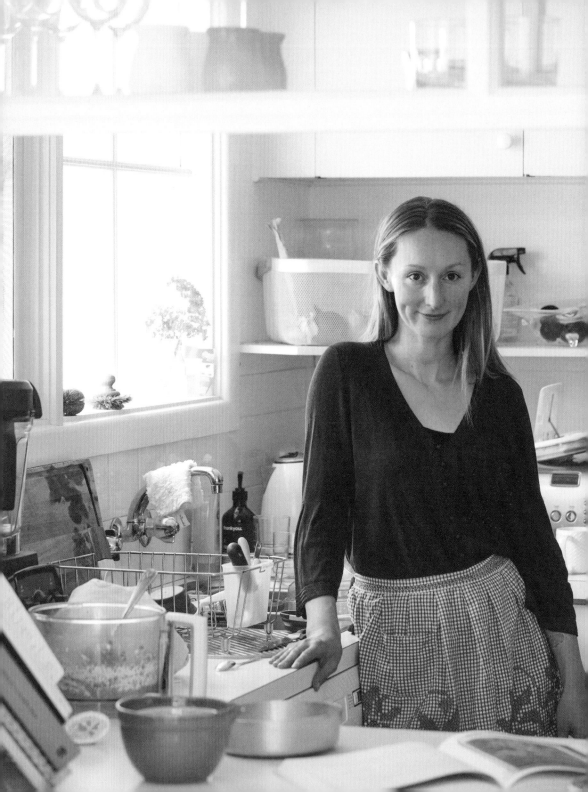

I cook and eat differently now that I am a mother. Before Joan was born I would spend great lengths of time in the kitchen – cooking to satisfy cravings and acquire culinary skills. Then I became the food source for a tiny human who was happiest in my arms all day and night. Suddenly, I needed things that were quick to assemble, easy to eat and nutrient rich; food that would replenish my body and fuel me through long days following sleepless nights. And so, I created a repertoire of meals to satisfy my new-mother needs.

Breakfast became eggs with avocado and my dad's sourdough bread. Sometimes I would serve the eggs over leftover vegetables or dhal; and at other times I would make something sweet – say, porridge (if I was craving warmth and comfort) or a smoothie (if I was low on energy). Lunch was invariably a colourful bowl of vegetables with legumes or tinned fish; or perhaps eggs on toast. Afternoon bites involved dates or a snack plate with sliced vegetables. Dinner would vary the most out of any meal, though we ate a lot of slow-cooked casseroles and simple pasta dishes.

To allow myself to eat in this restorative fashion with ease, I prepared as much as possible in the pockets of time when Ben was home and able to care for Joan. Eggs were boiled, oats were soaked, vegetables were sliced, quinoa was cooked and our freezer was filled with ready-to-grab meals. As the months and years passed, my needs, and those of my child, changed. I found myself once again having long blocks of time to cook and eat, and would flip through cookbooks for enjoyment and inspiration like I used to – only this time with Joan by my side, telling me what looked good.

My repertoire expanded, and yet I continued to favour an organised and replenishing style of cooking and eating. New-mother food is good food, and once I started eating this way, I didn't want to stop. So I haven't. Occasionally I'll cook something fantastical; and I still, of course, eat foods purely for pleasure (by that I mean I enjoy them without any regard for their nutritional value). But I also have an awareness of the way certain foods (like eggs, vegetables and dates, for example) make me feel energised – spectacularly so. Hand me one of Joan's 'chocolate clair' bars (page 276) and watch me glide with ease through the late-afternoon hours with a tired toddler at my feet and a newborn on my chest.

Things don't always unfold this way, I'll admit. Some days are simply a struggle. But with containers of roasted vegetables and boiled eggs in the fridge, and a freezer that is never without at least one serving of stock and dhal, I know I can always create a nourishing meal on the days I feel least able to do so. Incidentally, those are the days I need it most.

The recipes in this book reflect the season I am in. They are those I made as a new mother, which continue to nourish my family and me every day. You'll find my recipe for chicken stock, which fortifies our bodies and enhances the flavour of many dishes. You will also find the quinoa salad that seemingly gives me superpowers, and the beef casserole my daughter devours with more gusto than anything else (well, besides butter).

Good nourishment is, at once, crucial and challenging when you're a new mother. Thus I have made sure that the time you spend cooking these recipes will be worth it. Each meal and snack is terrifically nutrient dense, satisfying both your body's requirements and your eager appetite; and many of these recipes provide leftovers that can be incorporated into another meal. I have intentionally used the same ingredients multiple times, so you can use what you have on hand instead of having to buy more.

I hope these recipes serve you well, and continue to do so as your family grows, as they have my own. If any of the methods I use are new to you, know that they were once new to me, too. I encourage you to read through the recipe (both the ingredients list and method) a couple of times, then go forth with bravado. After a few attempts you'll likely gain the kitchen confidence you need to make the recipes your own.

You will see I have used garlic and onion in many dishes. If you like to limit these foods when breastfeeding, as some women do, feel free to reduce the quantity (though in many recipes I have already used less than I ordinarily would). Conversely, feel free to add more than I've indicated.

Some wedges of red onion would be a superb addition to the tray bake, as would a scattering of diced shallot in the salad wrap or over the quinoa salad. Remember that consuming garlic and onion (or any strongly flavoured foods) during pregnancy and when breastfeeding will give your baby a taste of these flavours, and may help them to be more accepting later on – so, keep that in mind.

Finally, a kitchen tip: set a timer. It's easy to get distracted at the best of times, let alone when you're in the new-baby haze. I can't tell you how many times I've burned a frying pan full of seeds, or put eggs on to boil only to leave them bubbling away for 30 minutes.

A note on ingredients

One lesson I have learned over the years is that simple, uncomplicated cooking relies on good-quality ingredients. When you use produce that has been grown in nutrient-rich soil and as the seasons intended (tomatoes and corn in the summer time, for example), little needs to be done to create a meal that tastes really good. The same goes for animal products; the flavour of stock made from a chicken that has had a happy life is better than from one who hasn't. Keep this in mind when you're gathering ingredients to make these recipes and others. As discussed on pages 184–5, shifting to a more sustainable way of shopping and cooking doesn't necessarily require you spend more money (sometimes it will, sometimes it won't), but it may require a change in habits. The taste of the produce alone will remind you it's a worthy change.

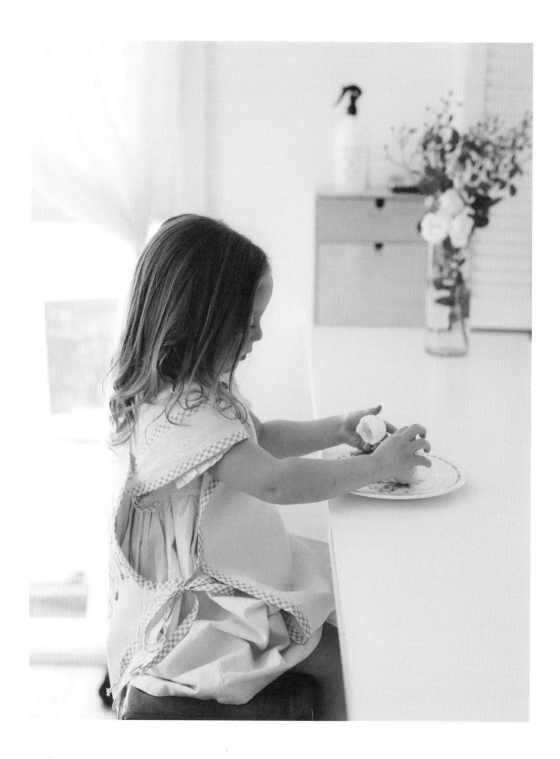

Fried egg and roasted vegetables

After Joan was born, I found myself gravitating towards savoury breakfast foods. A morning meal made with eggs and vegetables (and perhaps a scoop of leftover dhal or casserole) helped arm me against exhaustion – so much so that I would almost forget about coffee (almost).

Serves 1

½–1 tablespoon ghee (or extra-virgin olive oil or butter)

1 egg (or 2, depending on your appetite)

1 tablespoon sunflower seeds

1 handful of baby spinach leaves

sea salt and freshly ground black pepper

a sprinkle of chopped, fresh parsley (optional)

1 tablespoon hemp seeds (optional)

¼–½ avocado, sliced (optional)

ROAST VEGETABLES

1 medium-sized sweet potato, washed and cut into chunks

1 large beetroot, trimmed, washed and cut into chunks

extra-virgin olive oil, for drizzling

sea salt

To make the roast vegetables, preheat the oven to 180°C. Place the sweet potato in one roasting tray lined with baking paper and the beetroot in another, drizzle with the oil and season with sea salt, then give it all a good massage. Roast for 20 minutes and check for doneness (the vegetables will be cooked when the pieces are starting to brown and can be easily pierced with a knife). Shake the trays and return to the oven for a further 10–20 minutes as required. The beetroot will likely be done first and can be removed while the sweet potato finishes cooking. Set aside to cool.

To fry the egg, heat the ghee in a small frying pan over medium heat. When hot, crack the egg into the pan. Turn the heat to low and cook until the white is set. If you like a runny yolk, serve now. If you prefer a more well-done egg, flip it with a spatula and cook to your desired doneness.

Meanwhile, toast the sunflower seeds in a dry frying pan over medium heat until golden.

Place your desired portion of roasted veggies and spinach leaves in a bowl (storing the remaining veggies in the fridge). Serve the egg on top of the leaves, then sprinkle with the sunflower seeds, season to taste and add any additional ingredients.

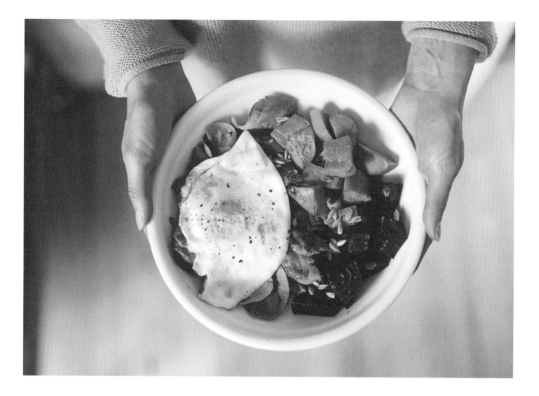

NOTE: *You can roast whatever vegetables you have on hand for this meal. Ideally, you will have leftovers ready to go. Roasting an extra tray of vegetables whenever you can – say, when you're making the tray bake on pages 298–9 – will mean you always have the makings of this meal in your fridge.*

NOTE: *If you wish to follow Ayurvedic and traditional Chinese medicine practices and avoid eating cold foods in the immediate postnatal period, heat leftover vegetables and leaves before consuming. You can do this in the pan alongside the egg or in a separate pot with a splash of water or stock.*

NOTE: *If you prefer, a sliced boiled egg from the fridge (made during a food prepping session) is a good substitute for a fried egg.*

Porridge with dates in ghee

This porridge recipe is one Ben took to making after I'd given birth to Walt. My friend Lucy, a recent graduate from the Ayurvedic Institute in New Mexico, gave me the idea of ghee-soaked dates when I sought her opinion on a porridge recipe using ghee (a prized ingredient in Ayurvedic medicine). Apparently, ghee-soaked dates are an ideal postnatal food, which is excellent news as they're also delicious – reminiscent of sticky date pudding.

Serves 1

½ cup (50 g) rolled oats

½ cup (125 ml) milk of your choice
   (I use organic cow's milk)

1 tablespoon sunflower seeds

1 tablespoon hemp seeds (optional)

pure maple syrup, for drizzling
   (optional)

GHEE-SOAKED DATES

5 large Medjool dates, halved
   lengthways, pits removed,
   then halved crossways

2 tablespoons ghee

¼ teaspoon ground cinnamon

⅛ teaspoon ground ginger

Place the oats in a container and cover with ½ cup (125 ml) water. Place in the fridge to soak overnight (see note).

To make the ghee-soaked dates, place the dates in a small saucepan with the ghee and spices, and warm the mixture for a couple of minutes over low heat until the ghee is melted and gently bubbling. Set aside.

Place the soaked oats in a small saucepan with the milk. Bring to a simmer and cook over low–medium heat for a few minutes, until the oats are soft and plump and the liquid has mostly been absorbed. Stir every so often to ensure they don't catch on the bottom.

Meanwhile, toast the sunflower seeds in a dry frying pan over medium heat until golden and fragrant.

To serve, spoon the oats into a bowl and top with the sunflower seeds (and hemp seeds, if using) and a spoonful of ghee-soaked dates. If you'd like a little extra sweetness, drizzle with pure maple syrup.

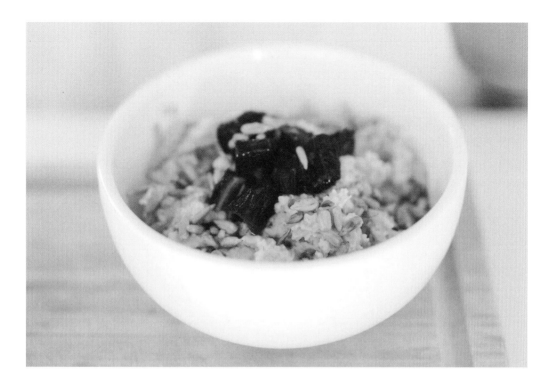

NOTE: *The recipe for ghee-soaked dates will give you more than you need for one bowl. Store the leftovers in a jar (on the counter or in the fridge – your call) and add them to your hot oats throughout the week, or simply snack on them as they are. Depending on your climate, the ghee will remain liquid at room temperature or solidify.*

NOTE: *Soaking oats can aid our ability to digest them. Personally, I am able to tolerate oats fine without this step, but I do appreciate the speed with which soaked oats cook, and find it makes for a creamier porridge. If you haven't managed to soak the oats overnight, you can still soak them in the morning shortly before cooking – even 10 minutes will make them softer and faster to cook. If you don't have time to soak at all, simply add ½ cup (125 ml) water along with the milk and expect it to take a little longer for the oats to cook.*

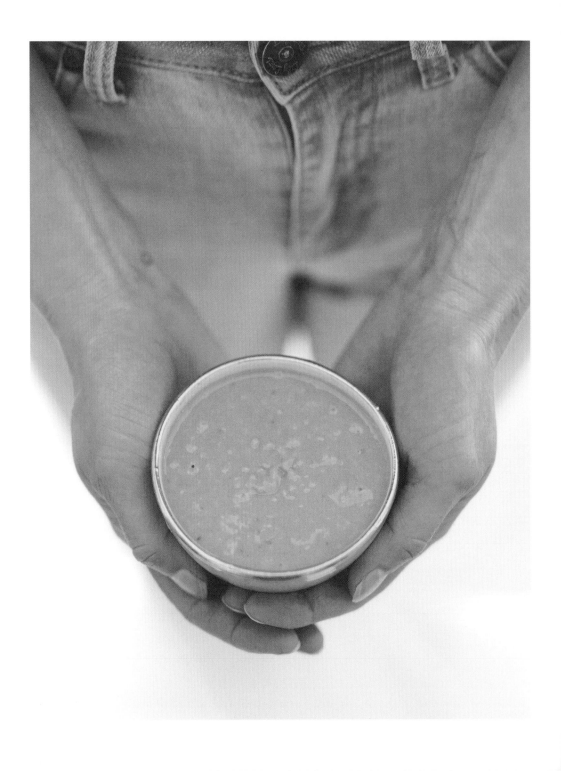

Hemp seed spread

Hemp seeds are one of my most used ingredients; I always have a jarful in the fridge. These tiny seeds, which are sometimes called hemp hearts, are fairly tasteless, yet highly nutritious, and can easily be added to most dishes. A tablespoon here and there throughout the day can quickly add up to a decent boost of protein and fat, which is handy if you've run out of eggs or fallen behind on meal prep.

One morning when attempting to sprinkle hemp seeds on my peanut butter toast, only to see them escape onto the plate, I had the idea of mixing the seeds with the spread before it met the bread. What resulted was a hemp-heavy paste that was dense in texture and nutritional value, and stayed put while I ate. No more chasing seeds around my plate!

Serves 3–4

4 tablespoons hemp seeds
4 tablespoons nut butter
   (I use unsweetened peanut
   or almond butter)

TO SERVE
sourdough toast
extra-virgin olive oil
sea salt

Place the hemp seeds and nut butter in a bowl and mix well to combine.

Serve spread on sourdough toast, with a drizzle of extra-virgin olive oil and a sprinkling of sea salt.

NOTE: *This recipe will give you more spread than is needed for one piece of bread. Store any leftovers in a clean container in the fridge to use over a few days. You can replace the nut butter with other ingredients, such as avocado, soft butter, ricotta or honey (even mayonnaise when making sandwiches), but keep in mind that some spreads, like avocado, are best prepared fresh.*

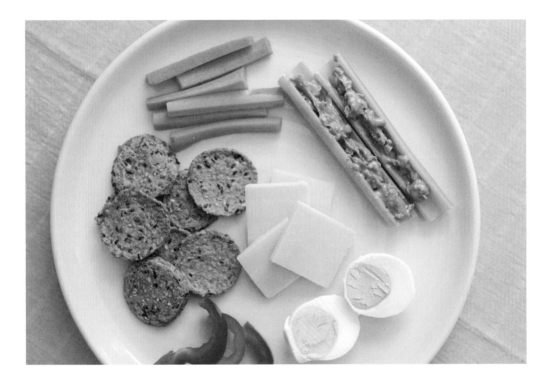

Snack plate

I love vegetables. Raw, steamed or roasted, I don't mind – I'll take them all. When Joan was a baby, I relied heavily on meal prep to get my vegetable fix. By cutting vegetables ahead of time, I was able to assemble a colourful snack plate easily and fill my body with more of the nutrients I craved throughout the day. Sometimes I would use green beans and snow peas, other times carrot and celery sticks. Many times I would actually forget to eat my vegetable snack, as I'd be busy staring at my newborn, so I would simply serve the pre-cut vegetables alongside something more substantial at lunch (such as tinned fish and extra crackers). This smorgasbord-type arrangement also makes a wonderful breakfast (similar to those eaten in Turkey – with little plates of vegetables, egg, cheese, bread and spreads) or dinner, when your freezer stores have dwindled and you simply cannot muster the energy to cook anything.

Serves 1

1 egg (see note)
sliced vegetables, whichever
   you fancy
cheese, hummus, nut butter
   and/or avocado
wholegrain crackers

To boil the egg, place in a saucepan and cover with cold water. Bring to the boil, then remove the pan from the heat and leave the egg in the boiled water for 7 minutes (for a soft-boiled egg, leave for 5 minutes). Remove the egg from the saucepan and place in a bowl of cold water. When cool enough to handle, peel the shell and cut the egg in half.

Arrange the ingredients on a plate or board and eat.

N O T E: *If you're boiling one egg, you might as well boil a few to have on hand. Boiled eggs in their shell will keep in the fridge for up to 1 week.*

Banana oat smoothie

When I was a university student, I would sometimes join Ben on his morning train ride into the city. Close to his office, and on the way to the library (which is where I would spend most of the day studying), was a juice bar. My standard order was the breakfast smoothie — a delightful concoction made with banana, milk and muesli. The muesli addition was, to my mind, ingenious, and inspired the smoothies I make today. Oats make smoothies thick and hearty, which is precisely how I like them. If you're in need of a pick-me-up, I encourage you to add a hefty spoonful of raw cacao powder to the mix, or shot of chilled espresso will also do the trick.

Serves 1

¼ cup (25 g) rolled oats

¾ cup (185 ml) milk of your choice
   (I use organic cow's milk)

1 frozen banana, broken into pieces

½–1 Medjool date, pitted
   (optional; see note)

1 tablespoon hemp seeds

1 tablespoon almond butter

¼ teaspoon cinnamon

1–2 teaspoons raw cacao powder
   (optional)

⅓ cup (80 ml) cooled espresso
   (optional)

This is an optional step, but if you would like a creamier smoothie, place the oats in a container and cover with ¼ cup (60 ml) water. Place in the fridge to soak for at least 1 hour or overnight.

Place all the ingredients in a blender and blitz on high until smooth. Pour into a glass to serve.

NOTE: *If you're not a fan of sweet smoothies, consider using just half the date, or omitting it entirely. You may not need it at all if you're using a plant-based milk, as they tend to be sweeter than cow's milk. You can also replace the date with honey, if you prefer.*

Green smoothie

If I'm not filling my body with eggs and veggies or toast in the morning, I'm often drinking a smoothie. Joan has had her fair share of smoothies in her time and is a harsh critic – turning her nose up at any creation that isn't adequately smooth or sweet. This green smoothie is one of her favourites. It's a source of plant-based iron, which is perfect for pregnancy, when our iron requirements soar. And thanks to the addition of kiwi fruit, it's also slightly tart – which, if you're anything like me, is also perfect for pregnancy (as I mentioned earlier, kiwi fruit was my number one craving when growing baby number two). Frozen mango is a nice addition, which along with the coconut milk will give the smoothie a tropical flavour.

Serves 1

¾ cup (185 ml) coconut milk (see note)
1 handful of baby spinach leaves
1 frozen banana, broken into pieces
1 green kiwi fruit, peeled
¼ avocado
1 tablespoon hemp seeds
½ cup frozen mango pieces
   (optional)

Place all the ingredients in a blender and blitz on high until smooth. Pour into a glass to serve.

NOTE: *I use coconut milk (from a carton) made with water, coconut milk, brown rice and sea salt. Coconut milk from a tin will work, though keep in mind it will create a smoothie that is thicker and less sweet. Homemade coconut, nut or oat milks would be ideal, although I rarely go to the effort myself.*

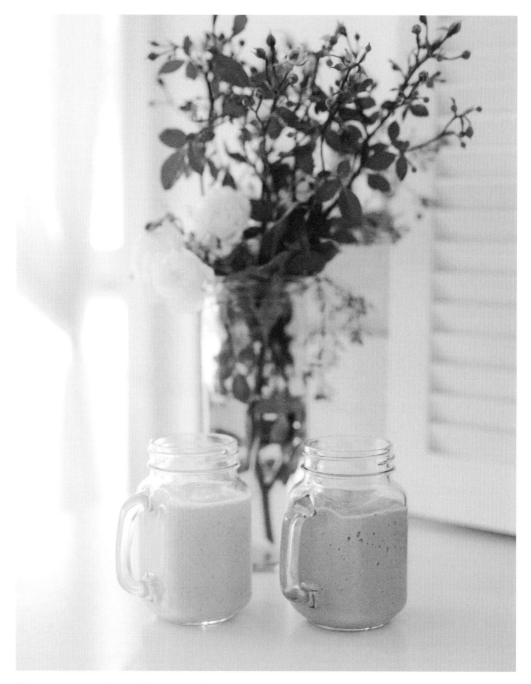

Banana oat smoothie and Green smoothie

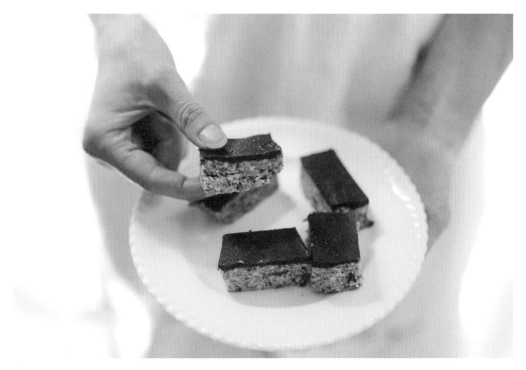

Joan's 'chocolate clair' bars

Joan's 'chocolate clair' bars

On especially tiring days, I'm grateful to have these bars in the fridge. Joan and I devoured batch after batch in the early weeks after Walt was born – each version slightly different. After the tenth batch, I asked Joan if she thought, as I did, that this was 'the one'. 'Yes!' she said, 'You should put it in your book.' (Bless her heart, she says that about everything I make.) I then asked her what she thought I should call the recipe, to which she replied, 'Chocolate clair.' It took me a few moments to figure out why she had chosen that particular name, as she doesn't know anyone named Claire. Then I remembered we had recently read one of her favourite books, The Lighthouse Keeper's Lunch, *in which the author makes reference to a chocolate éclair. Though these bars are a far cry from the French pastry, they do look somewhat similar – with their beige-coloured base and chocolate top. Regardless, I kept the name. It was just too cute to let go.*

Makes about 15 bars

¾ cup (115 g) cashews,
　plus extra if necessary
½ cup (80 g) unblanched almonds,
　plus extra if necessary
½ cup (50 g) rolled oats,
　plus extra if necessary
2 tablespoons chia seeds
2 tablespoons almond or cashew butter
2 tablespoons pure maple syrup
a tiny pinch of sea salt
4 large Medjool dates, pitted and
　roughly chopped
3 tablespoons warm melted coconut oil

TOPPING
2 tablespoons warm melted coconut oil
2½ tablespoons cacao powder
1 teaspoon pure maple syrup
a teeny-tiny pinch of sea salt

Lightly grease and line a 16 cm square cake tin or baking dish with baking paper.

Place the cashews, almonds and oats in a food processor and blend to a soft, fine breadcrumb consistency; some small chunks are fine, but don't over-blend or the mixture will get wet. Add the chia seeds, nut butter, maple syrup and sea salt. Combine the dates with the warm melted coconut oil and add to the blender (this will help to soften the dates slightly). Blend until everything is mixed together. The mixture should be moist but not soggy. If it's too wet, remove the contents and blend up some more nuts or oats, before folding them through the mixture. (Alternatively, you can add some almond meal, desiccated coconut, cacao powder or any other dry, flour-like ingredient you have on hand that you are happy to consume raw.)

Pour the mixture into the prepared tin, pressing down firmly with the back of a large spoon that has been dipped in water (this will stop the mixture from sticking to the spoon). Cool in the fridge for at least 1 hour until firm (to speed up the process you can pop it in the freezer).

Meanwhile, to make the topping, melt the coconut oil in a small saucepan over low heat. Sift in the cacao powder, add the maple syrup and salt, and stir until smooth (you may need to use a small whisk to remove any lumps of cacao). Pour the topping over the chilled base and allow to set in the fridge for at least 1 hour before cutting into bars.

Store the bars in an airtight container in the fridge for up to 1 week. If you leave them at room temperature, the topping will melt. Alternatively, you can store them in the freezer for up to 2 months, removing them 15 minutes before consuming.

Salmon smash

This wonderfully easy recipe offers an enjoyable way to consume more omega-3 fatty acids, which are so valuable in this season of life. The bones in tinned salmon are soft and edible, and a great source of calcium. Ben loves this salmon smash, as does my mother, who will add a scattering of capers to her serve.

This spread will last in the fridge for a few days and can be served on rye crackers, used as a sandwich filling or added to a snack plate as a dip for vegetables. It's also lovely stirred through cooked pasta shells or rigatoni, with extra parsley, lemon juice and some extra-virgin olive oil.

Makes about 3 cups

1 x 415 g tin pink salmon in spring
    water (with bones), drained
    (about 300 g final weight)
¾ cup (185 g) crème fraîche
1 large celery stalk, finely diced
juice of 1 lemon, plus extra if necessary
sea salt and freshly ground black pepper
1 small handful of fresh parsley leaves
rye crispbreads, to serve (optional)

Place the drained salmon in a bowl. Mash the fish and bones with a fork, then add the crème fraîche, celery and lemon juice, and stir to combine. Season to taste, adding more lemon or salt if desired.

Scatter the parsley over the top of your desired portion (storing the remainder in the fridge) and serve with rye crispbreads, or however you prefer.

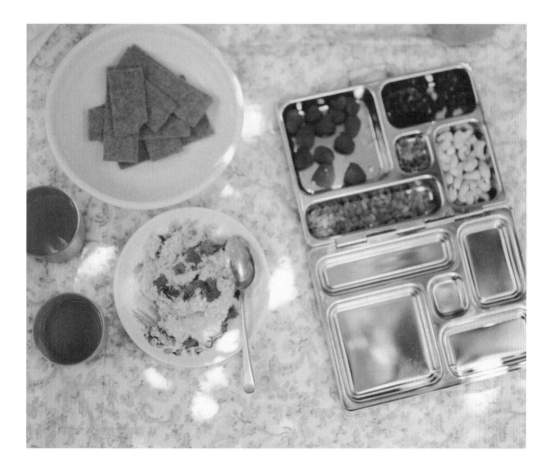

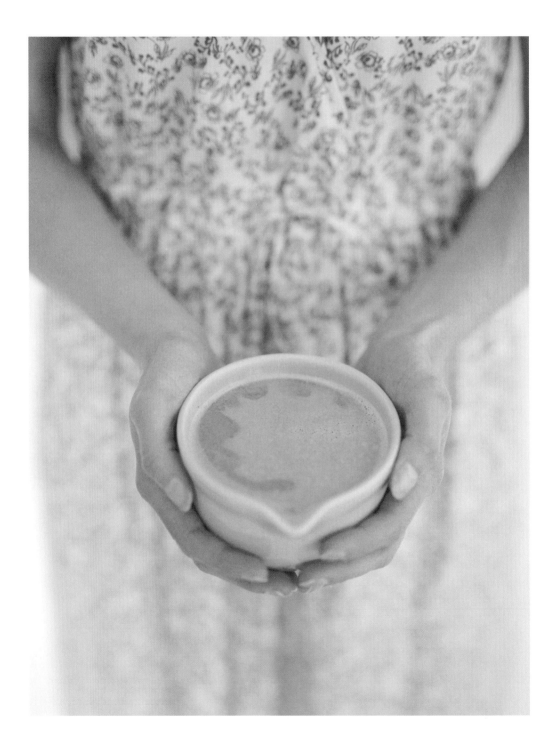

Hot cacao

There is something wholly restorative about liquid chocolate. On days when you're craving comfort (or 20 cups of coffee), this is precisely the recipe you need. While raw cacao contains only a fraction of the caffeine found in coffee, if you are sensitive to caffeine or believe your baby isn't a fan of raw cacao, you can leave it out and add ground turmeric instead, with freshly cracked black pepper to enhance your absorption of curcumin, a health-promoting compound found within turmeric. You can, of course, add the turmeric and pepper along with the cacao, if you wish. After my first pregnancy loss, I drank generous mugs of hot cacao with turmeric every day. It just seemed like a good thing to do.

Serves 1

1 cup (250 ml) milk of your choice
 (I use organic cow's milk)
2–3 teaspoons raw cacao powder
¼ teaspoon ground cinnamon
1–2 teaspoons honey
¼–½ teaspoon ground turmeric
 (optional)
freshly ground black pepper
 (optional)

Pour the milk into a small saucepan and place over low heat until heated through but not boiling. Remove from the heat, and whisk in the cacao and cinnamon and honey to taste.

If using, add the turmeric and pepper – start with a small amount and see how you like it before adding more.

Rainbow quinoa salad

This recipe includes so many of the foods I adore eating and that make me feel bright. I'll have one of these salads at lunch and, ideally, find myself soaring through the afternoon, caring for my dependent newborn and responding to my toddler's needs (and any tantrums) with ease. Note that I say 'ideally' – it doesn't always work out that way. But at least I will have nourished myself with a tasty meal. Take this recipe as a reminder to pause and feed yourself foods you enjoy, that make your body sing and give you the energy you need to care for your little one(s). Your bowl needn't always be as colourful as this – mine certainly isn't. As long as it contains veggies plus some sort of fat and protein, it'll do the trick. (Chocolate and coffee will help, too.)

Serves 1

1 tablespoon pepitas (pumpkin seeds)

1 handful of shredded radicchio
   or other salad leaves

1 handful of baby spinach leaves

1 carrot, grated (I use yellow
   and orange)

½ avocado

1 x 130 g tin salmon in oil (see note)

extra-virgin olive oil, for drizzling

juice of ½ lemon

sea salt

CHICKEN STOCK QUINOA

1 cup (200 g) quinoa, rinsed

2¼ cups (560 ml) Chicken stock
   (pages 288–9), vegetable stock
   or water

To make the quinoa, place in a saucepan with the stock and bring to the boil over high heat. Reduce the heat and simmer for about 7 minutes, until most of the liquid has been absorbed. Remove from the heat, cover with a lid and leave for 10 minutes. This will make more quinoa than you need for the salad. Store leftovers in an airtight container in the fridge and use within a few days. If you're pregnant, you might not wish to keep the quinoa for more than one day, and will need to heat it well before eating.

Meanwhile, toast the pepitas in a dry frying pan over medium heat until golden and fragrant.

To make the salad, place ½–1 cup of cooked quinoa (depending on your appetite) in a bowl along with the radicchio, spinach, carrot, avocado and salmon. Scatter the toasted pepitas over the top, and drizzle everything with extra-virgin olive oil and lemon juice. Add sea salt to taste.

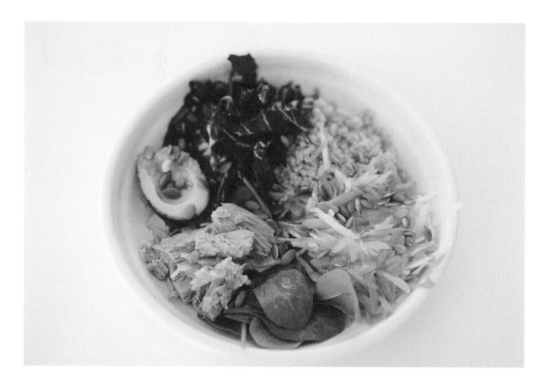

NOTE: *When adding tinned fish to salads, wraps and pasta sauces, I enjoy the flavour of fish that has been packed in oil (ideally, extra-virgin olive oil). You can drain the oil before use or keep the oil and add it to the dish — it's your choice.*

NOTE: *Try replacing the fish with boiled eggs, legumes or haloumi, or leftover chicken from the tray bake on page 298. A few pieces of the Quick-pickled beetroot on page 284 also makes a welcome addition.*

Salad wrap with quick beetroot pickle

After I gave birth to Walt, my midwife handed me a salad wrap, which I promptly devoured. Thus began my obsession with grated vegetables and cheese bundled into soft flatbread. If you can forgive the fact that salad wraps transgress the Ayurvedic and traditional Chinese medicine guidelines of having only soft, cooked vegetables and warming foods, you'll find them to be a great postnatal food. Not only are they delicious, they contain a variety of nutrient-dense ingredients and are easy to eat one-handed. They also come together quickly, particularly if you meal prep ahead of time or use leftovers for the filling. Better yet, have a loved one make it for you.

Serves 1

1 flatbread

½ avocado, sliced

1 small handful of shredded radicchio or other salad leaves

1 small handful of baby spinach leaves

1 small carrot, grated

¼ cup cooked quinoa (see page 282)

1 small handful of grated cheese

sea salt

QUICK-PICKLED BEETROOT

50 g raw beetroot (about ½ small beetroot), peeled and cut into matchsticks

whole spices, such as black peppercorns (optional)

⅓ cup (80 ml) vinegar of your choice (I use white wine vinegar)

1 teaspoon honey (optional)

To make the pickled beetroot, place the beetroot in a sterilised container or glass jar along with any whole spices you might like to add. Combine the vinegar with 1 tablespoon water and the honey, if using (you can use sugar instead of honey, but you'll need to warm the vinegar and water so it dissolves). Pour the vinegar mixture over the beetroot, cover and allow to sit for at least 1 hour before using. The beetroot won't pickle in this time, but it will adopt a vinegary flavour. Ideally, make the recipe and let it sit for 2 days before use. If you sterilise the container, the beetroot will keep in the fridge for 1 month.

To assemble the wrap, spread the avocado on the flatbread, layer on the remaining ingredients and top with some pickled beetroot. Season to taste.

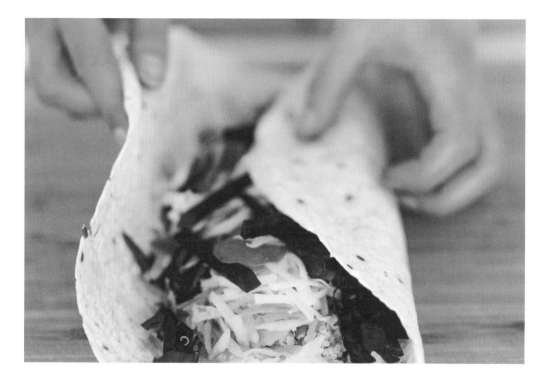

NOTE: *For extra protein, add boiled eggs, tinned fish or leftover chicken from the tray bake on page 298. You could also smash up some cannellini beans with the avocado to make a bean and avo spread. If you wish to skip the beetroot pickle, try sliced gherkins. Lastly, if you're in need of a more substantial meal (or if this simply sounds appealing), I encourage you to add some leftover roasted sweet potato (page 287) to your wrap.*

NOTE: *My family have been making quick-pickled vegetables for years – thinly slicing onion and cucumber, covering them in vinegar and storing them in the fridge for use in sandwiches. I favour beetroot as it adds bright colour and crunch; and, because it's one of Joan's favourite vegetables, she is guaranteed to eat it.*

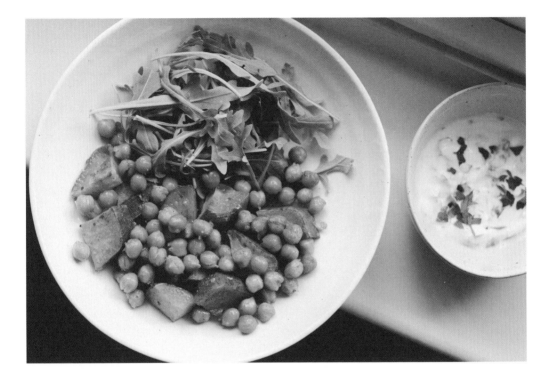

Roasted sweet potato and spiced chickpeas

My pantry is never without a tin of legumes. Black beans, cannellini beans, chickpeas and kidney beans – I like to have the lot lined up, ready to create a simple, nourishing meal at a moment's notice. Years ago, I started roasting chickpeas and adding them to salads. After spending time in a hot oven, the pallid chickpea becomes gloriously golden and incredibly moreish. The key is to dry them well before coating generously in extra-virgin olive oil. This recipe offers you another chance to use the garam masala and ginger you may purchase to make the dhal on page 293. You can also use leftover roasted sweet potato (page 264), should you have some in the fridge.

Serves 2

1 large sweet potato, washed
    and cut into chunks
¼ cup (60 ml) extra-virgin olive oil
sea salt
1 x 400 g tin chickpeas,
    drained and rinsed
1 teaspoon garam masala
1 teaspoon grated fresh ginger
2 handfuls of rocket or
    baby spinach leaves

YOGHURT SAUCE
½ cup (125 g) plain, unsweetened
    yoghurt (Greek or natural)
¼ cup finely chopped fresh parsley
1 tablespoon lemon juice
sea salt and freshly ground black pepper

Preheat the oven to 180°C. Line two baking trays with baking paper.

Place the sweet potato on one of the prepared baking trays and drizzle with half the oil. Add a small pinch of sea salt then massage it all together. Bake for 40 minutes, or until golden.

Meanwhile, use a tea towel to dry the rinsed chickpeas. Place the chickpeas on the other baking tray and sprinkle with the garam masala, ginger, a small pinch of sea salt and the remaining oil. Massage well to combine, then ensure the chickpeas are spread flat on the tray (i.e., not on top of each other). Bake for 25 minutes.

Meanwhile, to make the yoghurt sauce, place the yoghurt, parsley and lemon juice in a bowl. Give them a vigorous stir and season to taste.

Divide the sweet potato and chickpeas into two bowls with the rocket and serve with the yoghurt sauce.

Chicken stock

What food is more healing than a bowl of chicken stock? My freezer always contains at least one serve, which I will defrost and warm on the stove if Joan is feeling poorly, or we're craving soup, or simply to boost whatever it is we're cooking. Once you start making your own stock and using it to flavour your meals, it's hard to go back. Grains cooked in water taste lacklustre, and shop-bought stock just isn't the same (and the ones that might come close cost a fortune). This recipe will make a big batch that you can divide into portions and freeze, so you will always have a little liquid gold on hand. I sometimes like to add some chicken feet (you can get them from your butcher) to make a really gelatin-rich stock.

Makes about 6 litres

1 whole free-range chicken
  (about 1.6 kg), rinsed well
2 handfuls vegetable scraps
  (such as onion, garlic, ginger, carrot,
  celery tops, parsley stalks – see note)
a dash of vinegar (white wine or
  apple cider)

Place the chicken in a large stockpot along with the vegetable scraps. Fill the pot with enough cold water to cover the chicken, partially cover with a lid and bring to the boil over high heat. Reduce the heat to very low and let the stock bubble away for 45 minutes. At this point, keep the stock simmering, but remove the chicken and set aside to cool.

Meanwhile, skim the top of the stock to remove the foam that rises to the surface.

When the chicken is cool enough to handle, shred the meat and divide it into portions to store in the freezer. Return the bones and carcass to the pot, along with the vinegar, and continue simmering the stock for another 5 hours (or longer, if you wish). The water will reduce down quite a bit over this time, concentrating the flavour. You can top it up with water as you go, if you wish to extend the stock, though this will dilute the flavour.

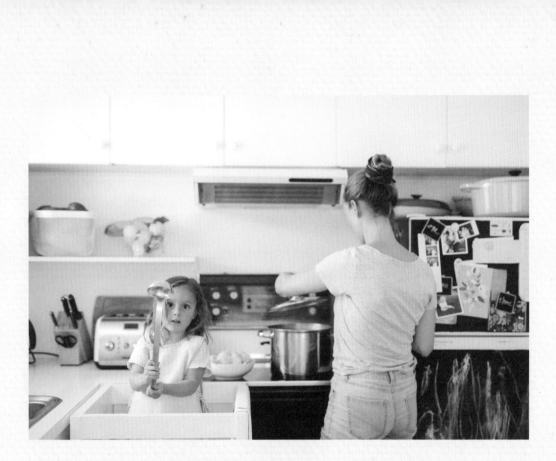

When your stock is done, strain it (discarding the solids) and store in the fridge for up to 3 days, or divide into portions and store in the freezer for up to 6 months.

Stock stored in the fridge will hopefully become gelatinous and develop a layer of fat on the top. Don't discard this when reheating – that's the good stuff.

N O T E: *This recipe is a great way to use up slightly tired-looking vegetables, and one blog reader encouraged me to freeze my vegetable scraps, such as peelings from carrots and celery tops, saving them for when you make a batch of stock. What a great way to reduce food waste.*

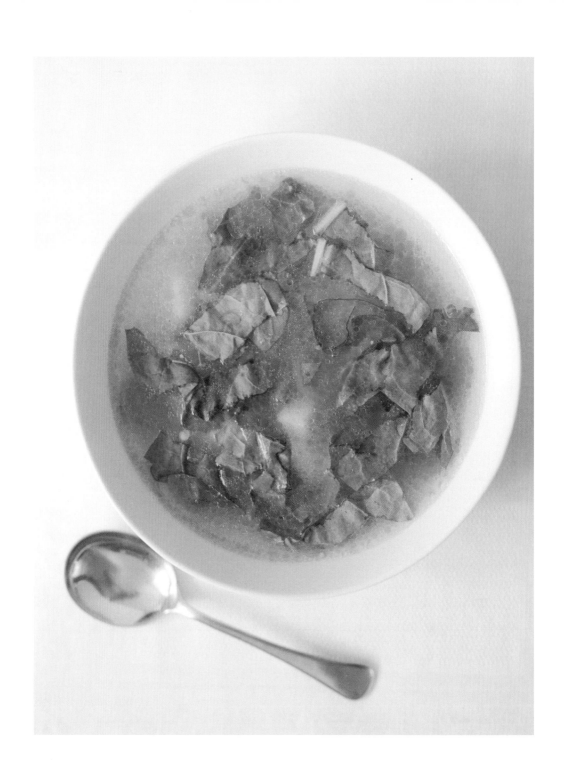

Flexible veggie soup

One of my family's favourite ways to enjoy our homemade chicken stock is in this soup. It's a humble preparation, with the deliciousness determined entirely by the quality of your stock. On the days I'm craving a bigger protein hit, I will add either shredded chicken (gathered during the stock-making process) or tinned chickpeas – but it's perfectly wonderful with just potatoes, carrots and greens. Nettle leaves make a nice addition and will give you a nourishing boost in the postnatal period (thanks to my friend Robin for the nettle inspiration). When making a big batch of this soup for either the freezer or to eat over consecutive days, I will take it off the heat before the vegetables are completely cooked (as I know they'll get a second heating).

Serves 2–4

1 tablespoon ghee
  or extra-virgin olive oil
½ brown onion, diced
sea salt
1 garlic clove, sliced
4 cups (1 litre) Chicken stock
  (pages 288–9) or vegetable stock
2 medium-sized waxy potatoes
  (such as Dutch creams), cut into
  2 cm chunks
2 carrots, sliced
1–2 handfuls of shredded chicken
  (optional)
1 handful of sliced silverbeet
freshly ground black pepper

Heat the ghee or oil in a large heavy-based saucepan over low heat. Add the onion and a pinch of sea salt and cook for 5 minutes until soft, then add the garlic and cook for a further 1 minute. Add the stock and potato, increase the heat to high and bring to the boil. Reduce the heat and simmer for 10 minutes, before adding the carrot and cooking for a further 5 minutes or until the vegetables are tender. If using chicken, add it in the final minutes of cooking to allow it to heat through. Just before serving add the silverbeet and season to taste.

N O T E : *If you prefer a plant-based soup, use a quality vegetable stock instead of chicken stock.*

N O T E : *Feel free to add whatever seasonal vegetables you wish (some chopped asparagus would be lovely in spring). Just be sure to add any faster-cooking vegetables at the last minute, so as not to overcook them.*

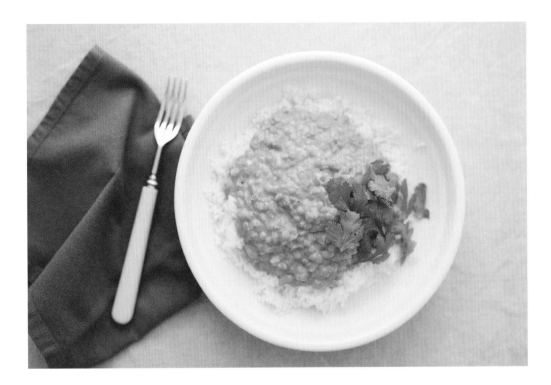

NOTE: *Be sure to use red split lentils for this recipe, not whole red lentils. Different varieties have different cooking times, and whole red lentils take longer to cook than split.*

NOTE: *Leftover dhal is lovely for breakfast with Fried egg and roasted vegetables (page 264), or added to the Rainbow quinoa salad (page 282) in place of fish.*

Red lentil dhal

I grew up eating dhal. Or rather, a tomatoey lentil dish my mother would call dhal. In reality, her version is more French-inspired than the dishes found in India and its neighbouring countries. Years later, I realised the reason we ate it so often was that it would readily, and economically, satisfy the appetites of three hungry children, especially when served over mountains of rice. Occasionally my mother would bake leftover lentils inside puff pastry – making a lentil pastie, of sorts (much to the delight of my brothers and me). Now, as a mother myself, I see with new eyes the way my mother nourished her family, and take great inspiration from it. Joan has been eating this recipe since she was a baby – cleaning her plate no matter how it's served. Like my mother's dhal, mine is non-traditional and completely satisfying.

Serves 6

2 tablespoons ghee
   or extra-virgin olive oil
½ brown onion, finely diced
sea salt
3 garlic cloves, crushed
1 teaspoon grated fresh ginger
1 teaspoon ground turmeric
1 teaspoon ground cumin
½ teaspoon garam masala
2 cups (400 g) red split lentils
   (see note), rinsed and drained
1 x 400 ml tin coconut milk
1 x 400 g tin diced tomatoes
2 cups (500 ml) Chicken stock
   (pages 288–9), vegetable stock
   or water
steamed rice, to serve
fresh coriander leaves, to serve
lime wedges, to serve
1 handful of baby spinach leaves
   (optional)

Heat the ghee or oil in a large heavy-based saucepan over low heat. Add the onion and a pinch of sea salt and cook for 5 minutes until soft. Add the garlic and ginger and cook for 1 minute, then add the spices and cook for a further 1 minute.

Add the lentils, stirring to coat them in the spiced onion mixture. Add the coconut milk, tomatoes and stock or water, and increase the heat to bring to a gentle simmer. Reduce the heat to low and cook for 15–20 minutes or until the lentils are soft, stirring the pot every so often to ensure the lentils don't catch on the bottom.

Serve with rice, coriander and a squeeze of fresh lime juice, and, if you like, a handful of fresh spinach leaves.

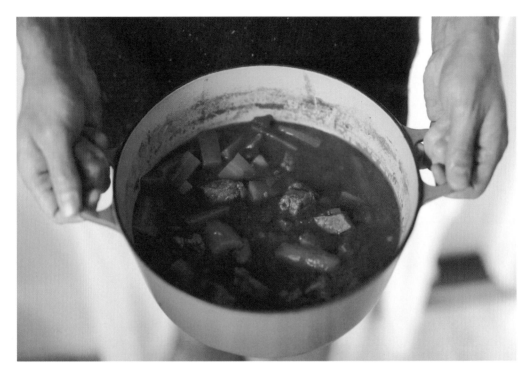

Slow-cooked beef casserole

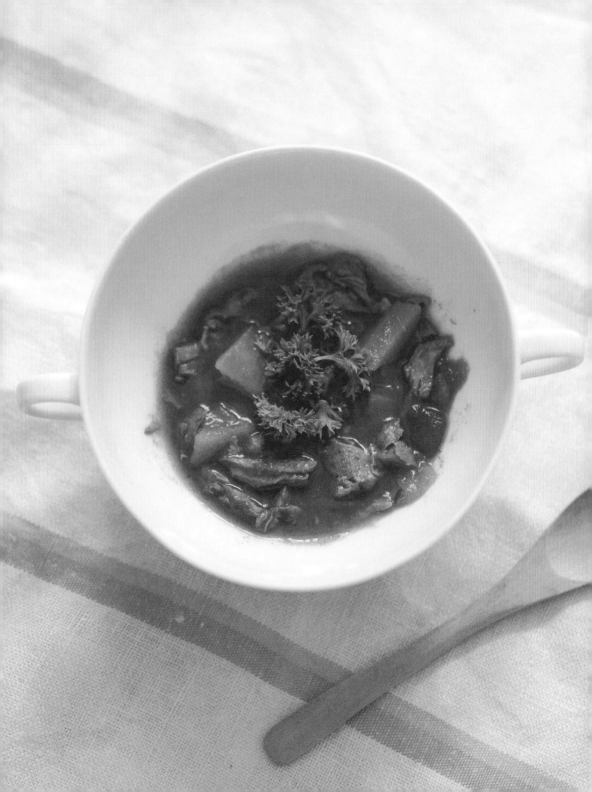

Slow-cooked beef casserole

If I had to name my family's best-loved recipe, this might be the one. We all perk up at the scent of it bubbling away on the stove. While Joan isn't overly fond of meat, she enjoys it when served in this manner. She prefers the carrots, though, which is why my recipe is so carrot-heavy – you may like to reduce the quantity and add some quartered potatoes early on, along with the stock and tomatoes. The key with this recipe is the long cooking time. I like to make this casserole a day ahead and allow it to sit in the fridge overnight – I find that the flavour only improves with time and the meat becomes even more fall-apart tender.

Serves 8

3 tablespoons ghee
   or extra-virgin olive oil
1 brown onion, diced
sea salt
4 garlic cloves, crushed
1 teaspoon sweet paprika
   or dried oregano
3 anchovy fillets (I use the oil-packed
   variety from a jar; optional)
1 tablespoon tomato paste
800 g diced stewing beef (I use
   chuck steak or beef cheeks –
   don't go for lean cuts)
4 cups (1 litre) Chicken stock
   (pages 288–9; see note) or beef stock
1 x 400 g tin diced tomatoes
5 carrots, cut into 6 cm batons
freshly ground black pepper
chopped fresh parsley leaves, to garnish

NOTE: *If you use shop-bought stock, it will likely be saltier than the homemade stock, so you might want to select a salt-reduced variety and use just 500 ml of the bought stock along with 500 ml of water.*

NOTE: *If omitting the anchovies, as I imagine some will (they're a divisive little fish), you may have to add a touch more salt. I encourage you to try them, though. They melt away, leaving you with a rich, salty flavour.*

NOTE: *You can serve this casserole however you like, with couscous, quinoa, rice, pasta or crusty sourdough bread – our favourite is on top of potatoes that have been boiled then mashed with butter and crème fraiche. It's sublime.*

Heat 1 tablespoon of the ghee or oil in a large heavy-based saucepan (I use a 26 cm Dutch oven) over medium heat. Add the onion and a tiny pinch of sea salt, reduce the heat to low and cook for 5 minutes until soft, then add the garlic and cook for a further 1 minute. Add the paprika or oregano, anchovies, if using, and tomato paste, then cook for 1 minute. Remove the pan from the heat, transfer the contents to a bowl and set aside. If you like, you can wipe the pan clean or, if you want extra flavour, leave the residue.

Return the pan to the stovetop over medium heat and add a second tablespoon of the ghee or oil. Brown the meat in two batches, adding a small pinch of salt with each batch and heating the remaining tablespoon of ghee or oil between the first and second batches. You'll get some browned bits on the bottom – that's good, they add loads of flavour – but if you feel the meat is catching or close to burning, you can deglaze by adding a splash of chicken stock and scraping the bottom of the pan with a wooden spoon. Once the second batch of meat is browned, deglaze the pan with a splash of stock, then return the first batch of meat and the onion mixture to the pan.

Add the stock and tinned tomatoes and stir well. Cover with a lid, leaving it up slightly so there's a small space for steam to escape, bring to the boil, then reduce to the lowest heat and simmer for 3 hours, letting it languidly bubble away. Add the carrots then cook for a further 2 hours.

Once the stew is cooked, you can serve it however you like, garnished with a little fresh parsley. Ideally, I like to let it cool completely and then pop the whole pot in the fridge to sit overnight. Then you can set aside portions for freezing and gently reheat the rest for your meal.

Chicken, tomato and potato tray bake

Arranging a bunch of ingredients in a tray, drizzling generously with olive oil and roasting the whole thing in the oven is such a rewarding way to cook. There is no searing or stirring involved – the food gathers a gorgeous flavour all on its own and, unless you're feeding a crowd, you're almost guaranteed leftovers that can be served for breakfast or in a wrap (see pages 264 and 284). Chicken thighs work perfectly in this sort of preparation, as they stay tender while you wait for the potatoes to turn golden. Once you've got this recipe down, try playing around with different variations. Slices of roasted red capsicum from a jar add a lovely flavour, as do black olives and sliced lemon.

Serves 4

5 boneless chicken thigh fillets

2 medium-sized potatoes,
    cut into 2 cm chunks

250 g cherry tomatoes

3 garlic cloves

1–2 teaspoons dried oregano

extra-virgin olive oil

sea salt and freshly ground black pepper

a splash of chicken stock, white wine
    or water, if necessary

baby spinach leaves, to serve

fresh sourdough bread, to serve

Preheat the oven to 180°C. Line a baking tray with baking paper. Place the chicken thighs skin side up (if using skin-on fillets) on the tray, spreading them open so they lay flat. Scatter the potato, cherry tomatoes and whole garlic cloves around, sprinkle the chicken with the oregano and drizzle everything with olive oil. Season well with a big pinch of sea salt and some freshly ground black pepper.

Place in the oven. Check after 40 minutes and spoon some of the juices over the chicken. If the tray is looking a little dry, add a splash of stock, wine or water. Cook for 1 hour in total, until the chicken is cooked through and the potatoes are golden.

Just before serving, scatter some baby spinach leaves over the tray, allowing the leaves to wilt just a little. Alternatively, place a small handful of spinach on each serving plate and top with the chicken, potatoes, tomato, garlic and pan juices.

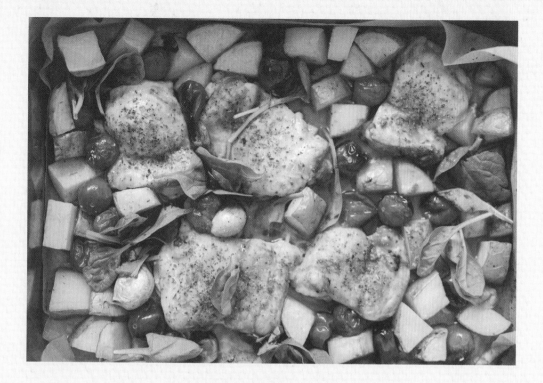

NOTE: *I highly recommend cooking a second tray of vegetables while you're making this dish, to have on hand for an easy breakfast or lunch, or to incorporate into other recipes.*

NOTE: *If you wish, you can replace the chicken with salmon fillets, sausages, haloumi or chickpeas. Simply adjust the cooking time accordingly and give the potatoes a head start.*

One-pot pasta with crème fraîche, lemon and peas

When Ben returned to work after parental leave, I tried my one free hand at one-pot pastas. This efficient and effective method instructs you to throw all the ingredients into one pot, allowing the pasta and sauce to cook at the same time, while cutting down your time spent at the stove and cleaning up afterwards. It's brilliant. The first few times you cook a one-pot pasta, you may need to supervise it closely to ensure your ratio of pasta to liquid is correct. But, like any new-to-you cooking method, once you've done it a few times, you'll gain confidence and can tweak the recipe to suit your preferences – adding some olives, sardines, cherry tomatoes, broccolini or whatever ingredients you fancy. In this version, I used homemade stock to flavour the pasta and provide additional nourishment.

Serves 4

3 cups (750 ml) Chicken stock
   (pages 288–9) or 2 cups shop-bought
   chicken stock
350 g pasta (see note)
1 small shallot, very finely sliced
1 garlic clove, very finely sliced
juice and zest of 1 large (or 2 small)
   unwaxed lemons
½ cup (125 g) crème fraîche
2 cups (310 g) frozen peas
½ cup (50 g) grated parmesan,
   plus extra to serve
⅓ cup (40 g) roughly chopped walnuts,
   toasted
1 handful of fresh parsley, chopped
sea salt and freshly ground black pepper

Add the stock, pasta, shallots and garlic to a large saucepan along with 250 ml water if using homemade broth or 500 ml water if using shop-bought stock (really, you can use whatever ratio of stock to water you want, as long as you end up with 1 litre of liquid in total). Bring to the boil over high heat with the lid partially on and cook, stirring every once in a while, for 9 minutes (see note), or according to the pasta packet instructions.

Meanwhile, combine the lemon juice and zest in a bowl with the crème fraîche.

About 2 minutes before the pasta is due to be done, spoon a couple of tablespoons of the pasta-cooking liquid into the crème fraîche mixture and gently whisk to combine, before adding all of the crème fraîche mixture to the pasta pot.

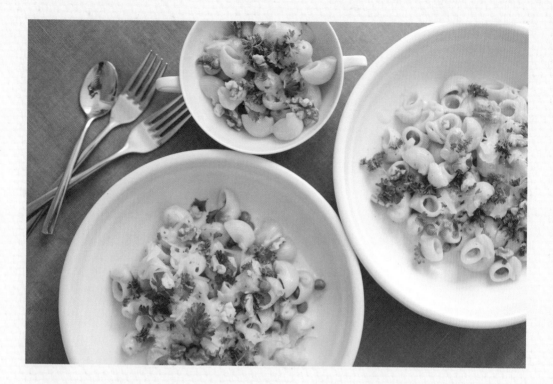

Test a piece of pasta, and if it is almost done add the peas. If not, wait another 1 minute before adding them. Add a splash of water if required, though go cautiously (you don't want to add too much).

When the pasta is cooked, stir in the parmesan then spoon into bowls. Sprinkle each bowl with the toasted walnuts, some parsley and extra parmesan. Season to taste.

NOTE: *You can use any pasta shape here – long or short will work. Just be aware that if you use long pasta you'll need a pot big enough for it to lie flat, and take note of the cooking time on the packet of your chosen variety: if your pasta takes closer to 12 minutes to cook, you may need to add an extra 125 ml of liquid. In this recipe, I used elbows that had a cooking time of 9 minutes.*

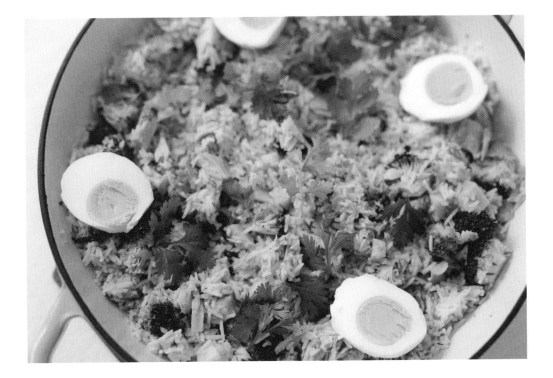

Kedgeree

This recipe is inspired by another of my mother's quick meals. I have fond memories of the two of us standing by the stove, talking about our day while she stirred curry powder and tinned fish into leftover rice. Every so often she would taste to see if she'd added enough curry powder, then sprinkle a little more until it was just right. Whenever I make kedgeree for my family, I am astonished by how tasty it is and how quickly it comes together – especially if you have leftover cooked rice. I add broccoli and stock to my recipe, and have replaced the Keen's curry powder with a fancier variety that is heavy on turmeric. Though good old Keen's works well, too.

Serves 2

1 tablespoon ghee

2 teaspoons curry powder

2 cups (140 g) finely chopped broccoli
(florets and stalk)

½ cup (125 ml) Chicken stock
(pages 288–9), plus extra if necessary

2 cups (370 g) cold cooked basmati rice,
from leftovers if available

a pinch of sea salt

1 x 185 g tin tuna, salmon or sardines
in oil, drained

juice of ½ lime

1 handful of fresh coriander leaves

2 hard-boiled eggs (see page 271),
cut in half

Heat the ghee in a large saucepan over medium heat. Add the curry powder and cook for 30 seconds until fragrant. Add the broccoli, stirring to coat it in the spiced ghee, then add half the stock and allow the broccoli to cook lightly for 1 minute.

Add the rice, salt and remaining stock, stirring well to heat the rice through. If it's sticking to the bottom, add a dash more stock or water.

Once the rice is hot, remove from the heat and stir in the tuna. Add the lime juice then taste and add more salt and curry powder if required.

Spoon into bowls and top with coriander and hard-boiled egg.

NOTE: *This recipe is really easy to make vegetarian: simply replace the tinned fish with tinned chickpeas and use vegetable stock instead of chicken stock.*

Yoghurt with toasted coconut and blueberries in maple syrup

Eating dinner early and breastfeeding a baby overnight means that, most evenings,
I fancy a hearty bedtime snack. If I'm short on time or energy, I'll simply take a spoon to
a jar of peanut butter and call it a day. Other times, I'll make this yoghurt bowl – with
tart, unsweetened yoghurt, toasted coconut flakes and blueberries, which I warm in a
mix of maple syrup and lemon juice (this combo is lovely over pancakes, by the way).
A balanced snack before bed will help keep your blood sugar levels steady, which can
reduce night wakefulness. That is, your wakefulness – your baby will still do his or
her thing. But at least you won't be ravenous while caring for them at 2 am.

Serves 1

½ cup (70 g) frozen blueberries
1½ teaspoons pure maple syrup
juice of ½ lemon
¼ cup (15 g) coconut flakes
1 cup (250 g) plain, unsweetened
    yoghurt (Greek or natural)

Heat the blueberries, maple syrup and lemon juice in a small saucepan over low heat until bubbling. Set aside to cool.

Meanwhile, toast the coconut flakes over low heat in a dry frying pan until golden (watch them carefully; they burn easily). Set aside to cool.

Scoop the yoghurt into a bowl then top with the sticky berry syrup and toasted coconut.

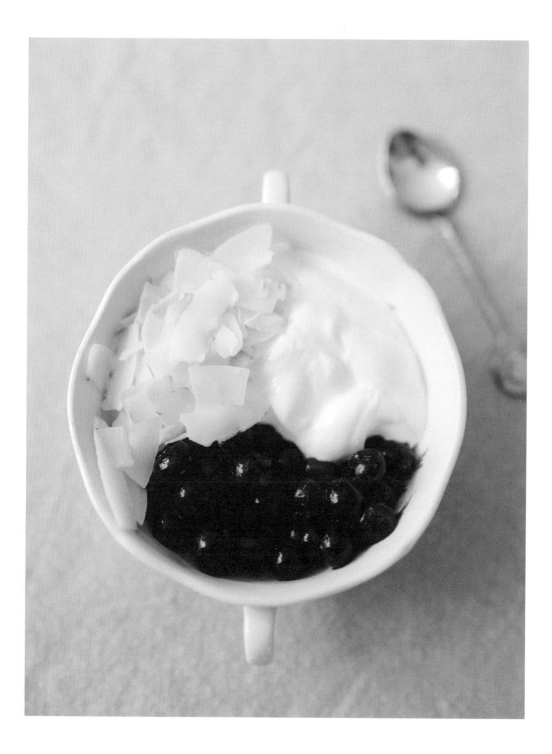

Acknowledgements

Whenever Joan achieves something that requires determination or gumption – be it buttoning a shirt, opening a package or riding a bike – she gets a certain look on her face. It's a look of joyful pride, of feeling super chuffed with herself. 'You did it,' I'll say, when her eyes find mine.

This phrase (which I started using after discovering the work of Janet Lansbury and Resources for Infant Educarers) helps her to become intrinsically motivated, focusing her attention not towards my reaction, but towards her ability, the process that got her there, and the fact that, yes, *she* did it. On her own! She stumbled, got back up and tried again, and gee it felt good.

Judging by the smile on her face, 'You did it,' seems to be just the thing to hear at the end of an endeavour. So I'm giving it a go.

I did it.

Week by week, as my belly and baby grew bigger and bigger, I sat at my desk in a nook in my bedroom and wrote this book. Sometimes the process flowed and sometimes it wouldn't, and yet for all that, I did it.

Do you know what? That does feel really good to say. The truth is, though, I didn't do it on my own. The story may be mine, but many people worked to get it out there. 'We did it,' is more apt, and I'd like to thank the people who contributed to *Nurturing Your New Life*.

Thank you to my agent, Emily Sweet. Without you, none of this would have happened. That you believed in me to write this book means more than you will ever know.

To the entire team at HarperCollins, thank you! Specifically to Mary Rennie, for your enthusiasm about the book's message and your support throughout the entire process – from proposal to pregnancy. I cannot thank you enough. And to Barbara McClenahan, for skilfully diving into the book and gracefully getting it to where it is today. Thank you to Hannah Koelmeyer for expertly editing the book and keeping the words grounded.

To Katherine Schultz, thank you for the most glorious photographs. You encouraged me to keep it real and captured the radiance within those real moments. Thank you also to Tim Grey for the photograph of me in my kitchen, content amid the mess.

To my blog readers, thank you for the time you've spent reading my words these past 9 years, particularly those of you who have been with me from the beginning. Thank you for consistently checking in and for your thoughtful messages.

To my clients, thank you for being vulnerable with me. To be your counsellor is a privilege.

To my friends, who went through the motherhood transition alongside me, thank you for your camaraderie, reassurance and snacks. You made this ride infinitely more enjoyable. Thank you also for listening to my book ideas and sharing your self-care stories.

Thank you to my mother-in-law, for the hours you spent with Joan so that I could write. Thank you to my dad, for the same, in addition to all our discussions on compassion and acceptance; the time you spent proofreading my work; and for all those loaves of homemade bread (keep them coming). And thank you to my mother, for the long days you spent at my home with Joan while I wrote, before going off to work yourself; for the discussions on mindfulness and motherhood expectations; for the times you would offer to come over at the last minute, just so I could get some more writing done; for the hours spent trialling and proofreading my recipes; and, lastly, for the way you mothered me. I wouldn't be the mother I am today were it not for you. In nurturing my brothers and me, you have created a legacy of connection, compassion and comfort that will undoubtedly influence the way my children parent their children, and then how they'll parent theirs. The impact of your love is immeasurable.

To my husband, Ben. Thank you for helping me create the space I needed to write this book. You are my greatest champion, and I'm grateful every day that you are my partner and that our children have you as their father. Thank you, also, for asking me to be your girlfriend back when we were 16. Let the record show I was only ambivalent until you held my hand. Then I knew.

And finally, to my children. First, to Walt. Thank you for being my writing companion those 9 months. The first couple were rough, but in the end we found our rhythm – me researching and writing while bouncing on a fit ball, and you wriggling about inside me. To write a book about growing new life when I, myself, was growing your new life was an extraordinary experience. Thank you for coming when you did. And finally, to Joan. Because of you, my love, I had a story to tell. When you're older, I hope you enjoy reading about our family when it was just you, your dad and me. Should you become a mother one day, know that I'll be there whenever you need me – to offer you nourishment, to do your laundry or simply to sit beside you.

Resources

Chapter 1: Tuning In

Mindfulness phone apps:

- headspace.com – Headspace
- smilingmind.com.au – Smiling Mind

Psychology resources:

- psychology.org.au – Australian Psychological Society website, for a list of practitioners

Chapter 2: Expectations and Compassion

Self-compassion research and resources:

- self-compassion.org – Dr Kristin Neff's website

Health at Every Size resources:

- haesaustraliainc.wildapricot.org – links to research on the benefits of a weight-neutral, non-diet approach and a list of practitioners, including dietitians, psychologists and personal trainers

Psychology resources:

- psychology.org.au – Australian Psychological Society website, for a list of practitioners

Report on the hormonal physiology of pregnancy and birth:

- nationalpartnership.org/our-work/resources/health-care/maternity/hormonal-physiology-of-childbearing.pdf – 'Hormonal Physiology of Childbearing: Evidence and Implications for Women, Babies, and Maternity Care' by Dr Sarah J. Buckley

Chapter 3: Support

Birthing books:

- *Gentle Birth, Gentle Mothering* by Dr Sarah J. Buckley
- *Ina May's Guide to Childbirth* by Ina May Gaskin
- *HypnoBirthing: The Mongan Method* by Marie Mongan

- *Mindful Hypnobirthing: Hypnosis and Mindfulness Techniques for a Calm and Confident Birth* by Sophie Fletcher
- *Juju Sundin's Birth Skills* with Sarah Murdoch

For anxiety and depression:

- panda.com.au – PANDA (Perinatal Anxiety and Depression Australia) supports women, men and families across Australia affected by anxiety and depression during pregnancy and in the first year of parenthood

Midwife resources:

- midwives.org.au
- midwivesaustralia.com.au
- eligiblemidwives.com.au

To hire a doula:

- douladirectory.com.au

For additional birth classes:

- au.hypnobirthing.com – for information on HypnoBirthing and a directory of practitioners
- calmbirth.com.au – for information on Calmbirth and a directory of practitioners
- shebirths.com – for those who want the option of an online birth course

For you and your partner:

- *Choosing Happiness: Life & Soul Essentials* by Stephanie Dowrick

Chapter 4: Self-care

Books I read to understand my child's development:

- *The Whole-brain Child: 12 Revolutionary Strategies to Nurture Your Child's Developing Mind* by Daniel J. Siegel and Tina Payne Bryson
- *No Drama Discipline: The Whole-brain Way to Calm the Chaos and Nurture Your Child's Developing Mind* by Daniel J. Siegel and Tina Payne Bryson
- *Elevating Child Care: A Guide to Respectful Parenting* by Janet Lansbury
- *No Bad Kids: Toddler Discipline Without Shame* by Janet Lansbury
- janetlansbury.com – RIE parenting resources
- The Wonder Weeks phone app – to explain the developmental leaps your baby is going through

Chapter 5: Sleep

For more information on safe bed-sharing and how babies sleep:

- rednose.com.au/article/sharing-a-sleep-surface-with-a-baby – Red Nose

Books for further guidance and support:

- *The Gentle Sleep Book: A Guide for Calm Babies, Toddlers and Pre-schoolers* by Sarah Ockwell-Smith
- *Sleeping Like a Baby: Simple Sleep Solutions for Babies and Toddlers* by Pinky McKay

Weaning resources:

- drjaygordon.com/attachment/sleeppattern.html – 'Sleep, Changing Patterns in the Family Bed' by Dr Jay Gordon
- *Weaning with Love* by Pinky McKay (available as a free ebook at pinkymckay.com/pdf/pinky_mckay-weaning_with_love_ebook.pdf)

Chapter 6: Nourishing Yourself, Part 1

Intuitive Eating resources:

- *Intuitive Eating: A Revolutionary Program that Works* – the fully revised 3rd Edition by Evelyn Tribole and Elyse Resch
- intuitiveeating.org – links to research and the book

Health at Every Size resources:

- haesaustraliainc.wildapricot.org – links to research on the benefits of a weight-neutral, non-diet approach and a list of practitioners, including dietitians, psychologists and personal trainers

Chapter 7: Nourishing Yourself, Part 2

Breastfeeding support:

- breastfeeding.asn.au – Australian Breastfeeding Association website

Fertility resource:

- tcoyf.com – Taking Charge of Your Fertility website

Chapter 8: Nourishing Your Family

Further baby-led weaning guidance:

- *Baby-led Weaning: Helping Your Baby to Love Good Food* by Gill Rapley and Tracey Murkett
- rapleyweaning.com – Gill Rapley's website and resources

Division of Responsibility guidance:

- ellynsatterinstitute.org – the Ellyn Satter Institute website

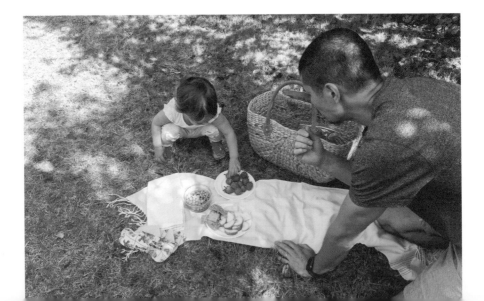

Index

Recipe Index